Gynecologic Pathology

Editors

BLAISE A. CLARKE
W. GLENN McCLUGGAGE

SURGICAL PATHOLOGY CLINICS

www.surgpath.theclinics.com

Consulting Editor
JASON L. HORNICK

June 2016 • Volume 9 • Number 2

ELSEVIER

1600 John F. Kennedy Boulevard • Suite 1800 • Philadelphia, Pennsylvania, 19103-2899

http://www.theclinics.com

SURGICAL PATHOLOGY CLINICS Volume 9, Number 2
June 2016 ISSN 1875-9181, ISBN-13: 978-0-323-44638-9

Editor: Lauren Boyle
Developmental Editor: Donald Mumford

Surgical Pathology Clinics (ISSN 1875-9181) is published quarterly by Elsevier Inc., 360 Park Avenue South, New York, NY 10010. Months of issue are March, June, September, and December. Business and Editorial Office: Elsevier Inc., 1600 John F. Kennedy Blvd., Ste. 1800, Philadelphia, PA 19103-2899. Accounting and Circulation Offices: Elsevier Inc., 3251 Riverport Lane, Maryland Heights, MO 63043. Periodicals postage paid at New York, NY and at additional mailing offices. Subscription prices are $200.00 per year (US individuals), $263.00 per year (US institutions), $100.00 per year (US students/residents), $250.00 per year (Canadian individuals), $300.00 per year (Canadian Institutions), $250.00 per year (foreign individuals), $300.00 per year (foreign institutions), and $120.00 per year (international & Canadian students/residents). Foreign air speed delivery is included in all *Clinics'* subscription prices. All prices are subject to change without notice. **POSTMASTER:** Send address changes to *Surgical Pathology Clinics*, Elsevier, 3251 Riverport Lane, Maryland Heights, MO 63043. **Customer Service: 1-800-654-2452 (US). From outside the United States, call 1-314-447-8871. Fax: 1-314-447-8029. E-mail: JournalsCustomerServiceusa@elsevier.com (for print support) and JournalsOnlineSupport-usa@elsevier.com (for online support).**

Reprints. For copies of 100 or more, of articles in this publication, please contact the Commercial Reprints Department, Elsevier Inc., 360 Park Avenue South, New York, NY 10010-1710. Tel. 212-633-3874; Fax: 212-633-3820; E-mail: reprints@elsevier.com.

Surgical Pathology Clinics of North America is covered in *MEDLINE/PubMed (Index Medicus)*.

Contributors

CONSULTING EDITOR

JASON L. HORNICK, MD, PhD
Director of Surgical Pathology, Director,
Immunohistochemistry Laboratory, Brigham
and Women's Hospital, Associate Professor of
Pathology, Harvard Medical School, Boston,
Massachusetts

EDITORS

BLAISE A. CLARKE, MBBCh, MSc, FRCP(C)
Assistant Professor, Department of Laboratory
Medicine and Pathobiology, University of
Toronto; Department of Pathology, Toronto
General Hospital, University Health Network,
Toronto, Ontario, Canada

W. GLENN McCLUGGAGE, FRCPath
Department of Pathology, Royal Victoria
Hospital, Belfast Health and Social Care Trust,
Belfast, Northern Ireland, United Kingdom

AUTHORS

RUSSELL R. BROADDUS, MD, PhD
Professor, Department of Pathology, University
of Texas M.D. Anderson Cancer Center,
Houston, Texas

MARILYN M. BUI, MD, PhD
Scientific Director, Analytic Microscopy Core;
Senior Member, Analytic Microscopy Core,
Department of Anatomic Pathology, H. Lee
Moffitt Cancer Center and Research Institute,
Tampa, Florida

ADRIAN CHARLES, FRCPA
Department of Anatomical Pathology, Sidra
Medical and Research Center, Doha, Qatar

BLAISE A. CLARKE, MBBCh, MSc, FRCP(C)
Assistant Professor, Department of Laboratory
Medicine and Pathobiology, University of
Toronto; Department of Pathology, Toronto
General Hospital, University Health Network,
Toronto, Ontario, Canada

DEBORAH F. DeLAIR, MD
Department of Pathology, Memorial Sloan
Kettering Cancer Center, New York, New York

BOJANA DJORDJEVIC, MD, FRCPC, FCAP
Assistant Professor, Department of Pathology
and Laboratory Medicine, University of Ottawa,
The Ottawa Hospital, Eastern Ontario Regional
Laboratory, Ottawa, Ontario, Canada

WILLIAM D. FOULKES, MBBS, PhD
Departments of Human Genetics and
Oncology, McGill University; Department of
Medical Genetics, Jewish General Hospital,
McGill University Health Centre; Cancer
Genetics Laboratory, Lady Davis Institute,
Montreal, Quebec, Canada

C. BLAKE GILKS, MD
Professor and Consultant Pathologist,
Department of Pathology and Laboratory
Medicine, Vancouver General Hospital,
University of British Columbia, Vancouver,
British Columbia, Canada

CATHERINE GOUDIE, MD
Department of Pediatric Oncology, McGill
University, Montreal, Quebec, Canada

MARK C. LLOYD, PhD
Staff Scientist, Analytic Microscopy Core,
H. Lee Moffitt Cancer Center and Research
Institute, Tampa, Florida; Department of
Biological Sciences, University of Chicago
Illinois, Chicago, Illinois

TERI A. LONGACRE, MD
Professor, Department of Pathology, Stanford
University School of Medicine, Stanford,
California

W. GLENN McCLUGGAGE, FRCPath
Department of Pathology, Royal Victoria
Hospital, Belfast Health and Social Care Trust,
Belfast, Northern Ireland, United Kingdom

EMILY E.K. MESERVE, MD, MPH
Surgical Pathology Fellow, Department of
Pathology, Brigham and Women's Hospital,
Boston, Massachusetts

ANNE M. MILLS, MD
Assistant Professor, Department of Pathology,
University of Virginia, Charlottesville, Virginia

GILLIAN MITCHELL, MBBS, RCPSC, PhD
Medical Director, Hereditary Cancer Program,
BC Cancer Agency; Associate Professor,
Department of Medical Oncology, University of
British Columbia, Vancouver, British Columbia,
Canada

JAMES P. MONACO, PhD
Lead Scientist, Inspirata, Inc., Tampa, Florida

QUENTIN B. NAKONECHNY, MD
Fellow, Department of Pathology and
Laboratory Medicine, Vancouver General
Hospital, University of British Columbia,
Vancouver, British Columbia, Canada

MARISA R. NUCCI, MD
Associate Pathologist, Division of Women's
and Perinatal Pathology, Brigham and
Women's Hospital; Associate Professor of
Pathology, Harvard Medical School;
Consultant Pathologist, Dana Farber Cancer
Institute, Boston, Massachusetts

**KASMINTAN A. SCHRADER, MBBS, FRCPC,
PhD**
Diplomate, American Board of Medical
Genetics; Medical Geneticist, Hereditary
Cancer Program, Department of Molecular
Oncology, BC Cancer Agency; Assistant
Professor, Department of Medical Genetics,
University of British Columbia, Vancouver,
British Columbia, Canada

PATRICIA A. SHAW, MD, FRCP(C)
Professor, Department of Laboratory Medicine
and Pathobiology, University of Toronto;
Department of Pathology, University Health
Network, Toronto, Ontario, Canada

ROBERT A. SOSLOW, MD
Department of Pathology, Memorial Sloan
Kettering Cancer Center, New York,
New York

COLIN J.R. STEWART, FRCPA
Department of Histopathology, King Edward
Memorial Hospital, School for Women's and
Infants' Health, University of Western Australia,
Perth, Western Australia, Australia

LEORA WITKOWSKI, BSc
Department of Human Genetics, McGill
University, Montreal, Quebec, Canada

Contents

Hereditary breast and ovarian cancer (HBOC) syndrome and Lynch syndrome (LS) are associated with increased risk of developing ovarian carcinoma. Patients with HBOC have a lifetime risk of up to 50% of developing high-grade serous carcinoma of tube or ovary; patients with LS have a 10% lifetime risk of developing endometrioid or clear cell carcinoma of the ovary. Testing all patients with tubo-ovarian high-grade serous carcinoma for mutations associated with HBOC syndrome, and all patients presenting with endometrioid or clear cell carcinoma of the ovary for mutations associated with LS can identify patients with undiagnosed underlying hereditary cancer susceptibility syndromes.

Lynch syndrome is responsible for approximately 5% of endometrial cancers and 1% of ovarian cancers. The molecular basis for Lynch syndrome is a heritable functional deficiency in the DNA mismatch repair system, typically due to a germline mutation. This review discusses the rationales and relative merits of current Lynch syndrome screening tests for endometrial and ovarian cancers and provides pathologists with an informed algorithmic approach to Lynch syndrome testing in gynecologic cancers. Pitfalls in test interpretation and strategies to resolve discordant test results are presented. The potential role for next-generation sequencing panels in future screening efforts is discussed.

Small-cell carcinoma of the ovary of hypercalcemic type (SCCOHT) is a highly malignant and aggressive tumor and is the most common undifferentiated ovarian malignancy to occur in women younger than 40. SCCOHT is characterized by deleterious germline or somatic mutations in *SMARCA4*. Given the striking morphologic and molecular similarities between SCCOHT and atypical teratoid/malignant rhabdoid tumor, we propose this should be reflected in a nomenclature change and that SCCOHT be renamed malignant rhabdoid tumor of the ovary. SMARCA4 (BRG1) immunohistochemistry is useful in diagnosis because there is loss of nuclear immunoreactivity in SCCOHT but, retention of staining in mimics.

Patients with germline *DICER1* mutations are at increased risk of developing a wide range of tumors, most of which are relatively rare in the general population. In the gynecologic tract, these include ovarian sex cord–stromal tumors, particularly Sertoli-Leydig cell tumor, and embryonal rhabdomyosarcoma of the cervix. In some cases, these are the sentinel neoplasms. DICER1-associated tumors may have distinctive morphologic appearances that may prompt the pathologist to consider an underlying tumor predisposition syndrome and therefore consideration of genetic evaluation in the patient and her family.

Emily E.K. Meserve and Marisa R. Nucci

Peutz-Jeghers syndrome (PJS), in most cases, is attributed to mutation in STK11/LKB1 and is clinically characterized by gastrointestinal hamartomatous polyposis, mucocutaneous pigmentation, and predisposition to certain neoplasms. There are currently no recommended gynecologic screening or clinical surveillance guidelines for patients with PJS beyond those recommended for the general population; however, cervical cytology samples must be examined carefully for cervical adenocarcinoma. It is considered prudent, when diagnosing a potentially PJS-associated neoplasm, especially in young patients, to note association with PJS and recommend referral for genetic counseling. Complete surgical excision after a diagnosis of atypical lobular endocervical glandular hyperplasia is recommended.

Deborah F. DeLair and Robert A. Soslow

This review covers gynecologic manifestations that may occur in rare hereditary syndromes. Recent advances in disorders, such as hereditary leiomyomatosis, renal cell carcinoma syndrome and tuberous sclerosis complex, are discussed as well as lesions that occur in von Hippel-Lindau, nevoid basal cell carcinoma syndrome, Cowden syndrome, Ollier disease/Maffucci syndrome, and Carney complex. Characteristic clinicopathologic features of each of these syndromes are discussed with an emphasis on the key features that enable pathologists to identify patients at highest risk for these diseases.

Bojana Djordjevic and Russell R. Broaddus

This article reviews the main tissue testing modalities for Lynch Syndrome in the pathology laboratory, such as immunohistochemistry and PCR based analyses, and discusses their routine application, interpretation pitfalls, and troubleshooting of common technical performance issues. Discrepancies between laboratory and genetic testing may arise, and are examined in the context of the complexity of molecular abnormalities associated with Lynch Syndrome. The merits of targeted versus universal screening in a changing healthcare climate are addressed. In the absence of comprehensive screening programs, specific tumor topography and histological features that may prompt pathologist-initiated molecular tumor testing are outlined.

Gillian Mitchell and Kasmintan A. Schrader

Genetic testing for a hereditary predisposition to gynecologic cancers has been available clinically since the 1990s. Since then, knowledge of the hereditary contribution to gynecologic cancers has dramatically increased, especially with respect to ovarian cancer. Although knowledge of the number of gynecologic cancer–predisposing genes has increased, the integration of genetic predisposition testing into routine clinical practice has been much slower. This article summarizes the technical and practical aspects of genetic testing in gynecologic cancers, the potential barriers to more widespread access and practice of genetic testing for hereditary predisposition to gynecologic cancers, and the potential solutions to these barriers.

Hereditary breast ovarian cancer and Lynch/hereditary nonpolyposis colorectal cancer syndrome account for most hereditary gynecologic cancers. In the absence of effective cancer screening and other preventative strategies, risk-reducing surgery in women who are known to be at genetic risk of BRCA-associated or of Lynch syndrome carcinomas is effective in significantly decreasing the lifetime risk of developing malignancy. Reflex genomic testing of high-grade ovarian cancers and reflex immunohistochemistry in endometrial cancers will lead to greater recognition of germline-associated cancers. Approaches to processing surgical specimens, the recognition and classification of cancer precursor lesions, and differentiation from their mimics are discussed.

Special Article

Digitization of glass slides of surgical pathology samples facilitates a number of value-added capabilities beyond what a pathologist could previously do with a microscope. Image analysis is one of the most fundamental opportunities to leverage the advantages that digital pathology provides. The ability to quantify aspects of a digital image is an extraordinary opportunity to collect data with exquisite accuracy and reliability. In this review, we describe the history of image analysis in pathology and the present state of technology processes as well as examples of research and clinical use.

SURGICAL PATHOLOGY CLINICS

Preface
Gynecologic Pathology

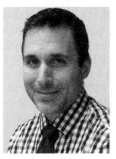
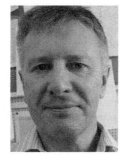

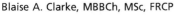

Blaise A. Clarke, MBBCh, MSc, FRCP   W. Glenn McCluggage, FRCPath

Editors

Molecular studies continue to validate and refine morphologic taxonomy of tumors and to explicate tumor associations. This is particularly true of hereditary predisposition in patients with cancer. With improved reproducibility in our assessment of ovarian carcinoma cell type, hereditary associations with specific histotypes have been established. Any patient with high-grade serous carcinoma of tubal/ovarian/peritoneal origin or serous tubal intraepithelial carcinoma should be referred for *BRCA1/2* germline screening given the high incidence of germline mutations in these patients (up to 25%). Patients with synchronous or metachronous cervical embryonal rhabdomyosarcoma and ovarian Sertoli-Leydig cell tumor were reported many years ago, prompting speculation that the co-occurrence of two rare tumors may denote an underlying syndrome; it has recently become evident that both tumors may be manifestations of the DICER1 syndrome, and their occurrence in the same patient almost certainly denotes the presence of this syndrome. Similarly, although familial small cell carcinoma of the ovary, hypercalcemic type (SCCOHT) was reported three decades ago, the underlying mechanism in both sporadic and hereditary cases of biallelic inactivation of the chromatin remodeling complex gene, *SMARCA4*, has only recently been elucidated; given the significant incidence of germline *SMARCA4* mutations in patients with SCCOHT, genetic counseling of these patients is mandatory. We need to be aware of the growing list of tumors, which, when diagnosed in a patient, should prompt consideration of an underlying syndrome and referral to genetic counseling services.

In addition to histotype-based strategies, reflexive biomarker-driven referral strategies to detect hereditary predisposition in patients with cancer are also becoming standard of care. Reflexive testing of endometrial carcinomas (irrespective of cell type and often irrespective of patient age) with mismatch repair immunohistochemistry is being widely deployed to detect underlying Lynch syndrome. In some centers, endometrioid, clear cell, and undifferentiated ovarian carcinomas are similarly interrogated, since we now recognize a histotype-specific association between these ovarian carcinoma subtypes and Lynch syndrome.

These laboratory-driven strategies address some of the system level barriers for genetic counseling referral, such as complexity of genealogy-based schemas and the poor implementation thereof, due to clinic visit time constraints and often the patient's unawareness of family medical history. Consequently, increased referral of patients to cancer-genetic consultation services is likely. There is also growing impetus for cascade testing of family members of patients found to have hereditary cancer syndromes, since screening and/or prophylactic surgery strategies in unaffected carriers have been shown to reduce morbidity and mortality in a cost-effective manner.

Increasingly, such genetic alterations transcend issues of hereditary predisposition and also convey therapeutic or predictive information, an additional catalyst for dissemination and uptake of such testing. For example, mismatch repair-deficient tumors may be targeted by immune checkpoint inhibitors such as PDL-1. PARP inhibitors are poised for clinical implementation, mandating *BRCA1/2*

Surgical Pathology 9 (2016) ix–x
http://dx.doi.org/10.1016/j.path.2016.04.001
1875-9181/16/$ – see front matter © 2016 Published by Elsevier Inc.

somatic and germline testing in patients with high-grade serous carcinoma.

In this series of articles, we highlight the critical role pathologists play in triaging patients for genetic counseling, either through the diagnosis of certain tumor types or through the reflex use of biomarkers. It behooves us as pathologists to be aware of these genotype-phenotype associations and to raise such issues in our reports, thereby directly impacting patient management. Cascade testing of family members is also yielding more prophylactic specimens from unaffected carriers, the assessment of which is critical and provides an opportunity for studying possible early or precursor lesions.

Molecular studies have not obviated histology but rather have underlined the critical importance of accurate morphologic diagnosis. The pleiotropic significance of an underlying hereditary disposition in patients with cancer is challenging how we implement genetic counseling, driving the need for clinically relevant turnaround times for these tests, and is changing the medical paradigm as we strive to balance "patient confidentiality" and "duty to warn" family members. Pathologists need to be cognizant of the diagnostic, prognostic, and therapeutic implications of these molecular alterations to determine how to deploy such testing and to ensure that, as testing algorithms become more complex and more dispersed, integration and interpretation of these findings with molecular-morphologic correlation and clinical contextualization occur.

As laboratory tests directly bespoke patient management, pathologists must be active members in the patient's circle of care, rather than relying exclusively on the vicarious pathologist-patient relationship mediated by the clinician. We need to reflect on the ethics of our technologies and consider the implication for the medical team of diagnosing or failing to diagnose hereditary predisposition in patients; this is something that has significant implications for both the patient and family members.

Blaise A. Clarke, MBBCh, MSc, FRCP
Toronto General Hospital
200 Elizabeth Street
Toronto, Ontario M5G2C4, Canada

W. Glenn McCluggage, FRCPath
Department of Pathology
Royal Victoria Hospital
Grosvenor Road
Belfast BT12BA, UK

E-mail addresses:
blaise.clarke@uhn.ca (B.A. Clarke)
glenn.mccluggage@belfasttrust.hscni.net
(W.G. McCluggage)

Ovarian Cancer in Hereditary Cancer Susceptibility Syndromes

Quentin B. Nakonechny, MD, C. Blake Gilks, MD*

KEYWORDS

• Hereditary cancer • BRCA1 • BRCA2 • Lynch syndrome • Ovarian carcinoma • Mismatch repair

Key points

- The ovarian carcinoma histotypes are different diseases, with different associated hereditary risk factors.
- Hereditary breast and ovarian cancer syndrome is associated with increased risk of developing high-grade serous carcinoma, but not other ovarian carcinoma histotypes.
- Lynch syndrome is associated with an increased risk of developing the endometriosis-associated ovarian carcinoma histotypes, clear cell, and endometrioid carcinoma.
- Screening patients presenting with ovarian carcinoma can identify previously undiagnosed hereditary breast and ovarian cancer or Lynch syndrome.

ABSTRACT

Hereditary breast and ovarian cancer (HBOC) syndrome and Lynch syndrome (LS) are associated with increased risk of developing ovarian carcinoma. Patients with HBOC have a lifetime risk of up to 50% of developing high-grade serous carcinoma of tube or ovary; patients with LS have a 10% lifetime risk of developing endometrioid or clear cell carcinoma of the ovary. Testing all patients with tubo-ovarian high-grade serous carcinoma for mutations associated with HBOC syndrome, and all patients presenting with endometrioid or clear cell carcinoma of the ovary for mutations associated with LS can identify patients with undiagnosed underlying hereditary cancer susceptibility syndromes.

OVERVIEW

Hereditary ovarian cancer syndromes have traditionally been underrecognized in medical practice and underreported in the literature. Recently, there has been growing awareness of the hereditary associations with gynecologic malignancies including ovarian cancers. There are 2 common autosomal dominant cancer susceptibility syndromes, hereditary breast and ovarian cancer syndrome (HBOC) and Lynch syndrome (LS), and both may present with ovarian cancers. In the past, the focus has been on breast cancers associated with the former and colorectal carcinomas associated with the latter. We review the epidemiology of these 2 syndromes in relation to ovarian cancers and the importance of accurate ovarian cancer histotype diagnosis in identifying these syndromes. Recommendations regarding the appropriate testing strategies for patients diagnosed with the high-risk ovarian carcinoma histotypes associated with the 2 syndromes, so as to identify index cases of these 2 syndromes and ensure patients and their families are able to receive appropriate screening and preventive treatment, are discussed.

Most cases of ovarian cancer associated with hereditary susceptibility are due to the autosomal dominant hereditary cancer syndromes HBOC

Disclosure Statement: The authors have nothing to disclose.
Department of Pathology and Laboratory Medicine, Vancouver General Hospital, University of British Columbia, Room 1200, 1st Floor JPPN, 855 West 10th Avenue, Vancouver, British Columbia V5Z 1M9, Canada
* Corresponding author.
E-mail address: Blake.Gilks@vch.ca

Surgical Pathology 9 (2016) 189–199
http://dx.doi.org/10.1016/j.path.2016.01.003

and LS. The role of pathologists in identifying patients with these syndromes at the time of ovarian cancer diagnosis is reviewed. An awareness of the ovarian carcinoma histotypes that are associated with these 2 cancer syndromes is of critical importance clinically and criteria for accurate diagnosis of ovarian carcinoma histotypes, their associations with HBOC and LS, and the clinical features of these syndromes, are presented in this review.

OVARIAN CARCINOMA

The World Health Organization (WHO) has reclassified ovarian carcinomas (formerly referred to as surface epithelial-stromal carcinomas) into 5 histotypes: high-grade serous carcinoma, low-grade serous carcinoma, clear cell carcinoma, endometrioid carcinoma, and mucinous carcinoma.[1] Each of these carcinomas is distinct in its histogenesis, molecular abnormalities, presentation, and outcome. The ability of pathologists to reproducibly diagnose each histotype has improved remarkably over the past decade,[2,3] with increased understanding of the morphologic features, immunohistochemical profile, and molecular characteristics, and this, in turn, has created opportunities for improved recognition of patients whose ovarian carcinoma is a manifestation of HBOC or LS.

HIGH-GRADE SEROUS CARCINOMA

High-grade serous carcinoma (HGSC) accounts for 225,000 new cancers annually worldwide and 140,000 deaths.[4] HGSC is the most common ovarian carcinoma histotype (68%) and accounts for a disproportionate amount of the morbidity and mortality associated with ovarian cancer. Recently, our understanding of this cancer has undergone very significant modifications. Serous carcinoma was formerly divided into low-grade, intermediate-grade, and high-grade groups (grade 1–3, respectively), but in the revised WHO classification, serous carcinomas are divided into low-grade serous carcinoma and high-grade serous carcinoma.[1,5] It must be emphasized that low-grade and high-grade serous carcinomas are not part of a continuum of disease, with an arbitrary cut point between the low-grade and high-grade cancers and frequent progression from low-grade to high-grade. They are 2 distinct cancers and differ with respect to clinical, morphologic, and molecular characteristics. It is also possible to reproducibly distinguish between them in practice, and this distinction does have clinical implications, including differences in association with hereditary cancer syndromes. HGSC

architecturally shows papillary, solid, and gland formation, with these architectural patterns frequently coexisting in a tumor. Indeed, the variability in tumor architecture (intratumoral heterogeneity) is characteristic of this tumor type, and reflects the underlying molecular abnormalities. The tumor cells consistently show high-grade nuclear features, with pleomorphism and a high mitotic rate and frequent abnormal mitotic figures.

Comprehensive profiling of HGSC through The Cancer Genome Atlas project has revealed that *TP53* mutations are ubiquitous, being present in more than 95% of cases.[6] *BRCA1* or *BRCA2* are also mutated or expression is lost through promoter methylation (*BRCA1*) in approximately 40% of cases. Apart from these mutations, however, there are few recurrent mutations in HGSC, which are characterized by chromosomal instability and aneuploidy, which leads to rapid accumulation of a wide range of structural abnormalities throughout the genome. There are frequent defects in DNA repair through homologous recombination. During tumor progression and spread, there is a high degree of intratumoral genetic heterogeneity, such that in samples from 4 different sites, in a single patient, only 50% of genetic abnormalities will be found in all 4 samples.[7] The mutant *TP53* is reflected in abnormal p53 immunostaining in most cases, manifest as either greater than 80% of cells showing intense nuclear staining or complete loss pattern, with no staining of tumor cell nuclei.[8] Any degree of immunostaining for p53 between these extremes of "all or nothing" is wild-type staining pattern and reflects an intact *TP53* gene.

Our understanding regarding site of origin of HGSC has also changed dramatically in recent years.[9] Formerly, based on the dominant mass theory, which assigned primary site based on the largest mass, most HGSCs were considered primary ovarian tumors, albeit with bilateral ovarian involvement in most cases. Very few cases were thought to have arisen from the fallopian tubes based on the formerly used criteria. The presumed histogenesis was of ovarian surface epithelium, which is of mesothelial derivation, undergoing Müllerian metaplastic change to tubal-type epithelium. Neoplastic changes then took place as a result of trauma and inflammation during ovulation.[10,11] One weakness of this theory was the lack of a recognizable precursor lesion. There is now overwhelming evidence that most HGSCs arise from the epithelium of the fallopian tubes and specifically the fimbriated or distal portion.[9] The in situ lesion, and earliest detectable manifestation of HGSC, is serous tubal intraepithelial carcinoma (STIC) (**Fig. 1**). Although apparently in situ,

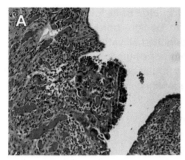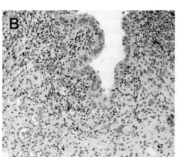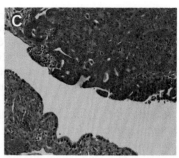

Fig. 1. (*A*) STIC is the precursor of most HGSCs, and is diagnosed based on the presence of cells with high-grade nuclear atypia replacing normal fallopian tube epithelium (H&E, 100×). (*B*) The cells of STIC characteristically show abnormal p53 expression on immunostaining; in this case, complete absence of p53 expression (p53, 200×). (*C*) The associated invasive HGSC is composed of the same cells, with poorly formed glandular spaces. Fifteen percent to 20% of patients presenting with HGSC of tubo-ovarian origin will have HBOC syndrome if tested (H&E, 100×).

STICs can be associated with transcoelomic spread and advanced-stage disease, even in the absence of invasion into the lamina propria of the fallopian tube.[12]

LOW-GRADE SEROUS CARCINOMA

Low-grade serous carcinoma (LGSC) has only recently been recognized as a distinct ovarian carcinoma histotype.[13] LGSC accounts for 3% of ovarian carcinomas. LGSCs are related clinically, morphologically, and genetically to serous borderline tumors, and in approximately half of LGSCs, there is coexistent serous borderline tumor. LGSCs tend to present with bilateral ovarian involvement and high-stage disease. LGSCs are believed to arise in the ovary, from serous borderline tumor (SBT). Most LGSCs show a distinctly papillary architecture, although some may be cribriform, and a variety of patterns of invasion by tumor cells may be seen, including single infiltrating cells, small nests of cells with irregular shapes, micropapillae, and macropapillae.[14] Necrosis is uncommon and psammoma bodies may be conspicuous. The nuclear features are lower grade than HGSC, with less than threefold variation in nuclear size. The nuclear features are similar to those seen in serous borderline tumors. Mitotic figures are relatively inconspicuous. LGSCs typically show wild-type staining for p53, reflecting the absence of *TP53* mutations. Clinically, women with LGSC present 10 years earlier than those with HGSC.[15] In common with serous borderline tumors, LGSCs frequently have mutations in *KRAS* and *BRAF* (in 50%–60% of cases). There are few chromosomal abnormalities in LGSCs in sharp contrast with HGSCs, and most are diploid or near diploid. The prognosis for stage 1 LGSC is excellent and surgery alone is effective treatment. LGSCs do not respond as well to platinum-based therapy as

HGSCs[16–18] and with long-term follow-up, most patients with stage III LGSC will die of disease.[19]

CLEAR CELL CARCINOMA

Clear cell carcinoma of the ovary (CCC) is the second most common histotype of ovarian carcinoma in Western populations (12%)[20] and it has a higher relative incidence in Japan, given that HGSC is not as common in Japan as in North America and Europe. The typical presentation of CCC is with low-stage, unilateral ovarian involvement, at a mean age of 55 years. CCC is strongly associated with endometriosis.[21,22] It is thought that CCC arises from endometriosis through a premalignant precursor lesion, atypical endometriosis, characterized by epithelial cells with moderate to marked atypia lining an endometriotic cyst, without evidence of invasive carcinoma. Architectural features seen within CCC include tubulocystic, papillary, and solid patterns. The identification of these architectural features is essential to correctly diagnose CCC, as many other cancers can display malignant cells with clear cytoplasm, and some of these have been erroneously diagnosed as CCC in the past. The cytologic features seen within CCC include cells with a cuboidal or hobnail appearance. The cells of CCC can be clear or have abundant eosinophilic cytoplasm (the oxyphilic variant of CCC). Other less common histologic features of CCC include intracytoplasmic hyaline globules, intracystic mucin, colloidlike material, signet ring cells (rarely), or occasional psammoma bodies. CCC may be associated with endometriosis, an adenofibromatous component, or both. Dense hyaline accumulations within the stroma of the papillary structures are a very helpful diagnostic feature, as this is not a finding in other ovarian carcinoma histotypes.

Molecular abnormalities identified within CCC include mutations in *ARID1A* (which encodes BAF250A, a subunit of the SWI/SNF chromatin remodeling complex),[23,24] *PIK3CA*,[25–27] and *PTEN*,[28] as well as microsatellite instability/abnormal expression of DNA mismatch repair enzymes.[29–31]

Stage Ia CCC has an excellent prognosis, whereas cancers that are higher stage have a poor prognosis. CCC typically does not respond to platinum-based chemotherapy, but may be responsive to radiotherapy.[32–34]

ENDOMETRIOID CARCINOMA

Endometrioid carcinoma (EC) is the third most common histotype of ovarian epithelial carcinomas. Similar to CCC, a large proportion of ECs are associated with endometriosis either within the ovary or elsewhere in the pelvis.[35,36] The average age of women with EC is 58 and women with associated endometriosis are on average 5 to 10 years younger when they develop ovarian carcinoma as compared with those women without endometriosis.[37] Women with EC may be asymptomatic whereas others present with symptoms related to their pelvic mass. Endometrial carcinoma occurs concurrently in 20% or more of the cases of ovarian EC.[38–40]

EC arises from endometriosis that has undergone hyperplasia and changes that are morphologically indistinguishable from atypical hyperplasia of eutopic endometrium. EC shows similar histologic features to those seen in the more common endometrioid carcinomas of the endometrium, including frequent squamous metaplasia, villoglandular architecture, secretory changes, oxyphilic variant, and sex cord-stromal-like architecture.

The molecular abnormalities in EC include inactivating mutations in the *PTEN* gene,[41,42] B-catenin-mediated canonical Wnt pathway signal dysregulation,[43–46] and inactivating mutations of *ARID1A*, which is identified in up to 30% of EC.[24]

MUCINOUS CARCINOMA

Primary mucinous carcinomas (MC) of the ovary accounts for 3% to 4% of all primary ovarian epithelial carcinomas. The mean age at presentation is 45 years[1] and most tumors are stage Ia at presentation.[47] When MC recurs, it tends to recur early and does not respond well to either radiation therapy or chemotherapy.[48] MC often arises from a borderline tumor or less commonly in association with a teratoma; these latter tumors are of germ cell origin, based on genetic analyses, whereas those without an associated teratoma

are not.[49] Often a range of histologic findings can be identified with benign, borderline, and malignant features identified all within one section.

The most common mutation molecular abnormality in MC is mutations in *KRAS*.[50–53] *HER2* amplification is identified in 15% to 20% of cases.[54]

OVARIAN CARCINOMA: HISTOTYPE DIFFERENTIAL DIAGNOSIS

Given the importance of accurate histotype diagnosis in assessment of risk of an underlying hereditary cancer syndrome, it is important to be aware of the common problems encountered in differential diagnosis.

- *HGSC versus EC*: It has been recognized that many tumors previously classified as high-grade EC primarily because of glandular architecture are now best classified as HGSC. Several studies have shown that the gene expression profiles of many of these cancers previously diagnosed as high-grade EC are identical to high-grade SC[55,56] and abnormal p53 expression and WT1 expression, features of HGSC, are frequently identified. Finally, high-grade EC does not typically have the same genetic mutations characteristic of low-grade EC, such as inactivating mutations in *PTEN*,[41,42] *B-catenin*,[43–46,56] and *ARID1A*,[24] indicating that they have not arisen through progression of low-grade EC. High-grade EC does exist but is uncommon (fewer than 1% of ovarian carcinomas) and can best be identified in practice by the presence of a low-grade component or squamous metaplasia.
- *HGSC versus CCC*: Although clear cells can be seen in HGSC, other more typical areas are almost invariably present, and facilitate arriving at a correct diagnosis. In difficult cases, immunostaining will help, as CCC and HGSC have different immunoprofiles; CCCs are typically WT-1 negative, estrogen receptor-negative, and positive for HNF1-b and NapsinA expression.[57] p53 is wild type in most CCCs.
- *HGSC versus LGSC*: The differential diagnosis between HGSC and LGSC is straightforward in most instances, with the former showing nuclear pleomorphism and the latter uniform tumor cell nuclei (less than threefold variation in nuclear size). In problematic cases, mitotic activity (fewer than 14 mitotic figures per 10 high-power fields) or wild-type staining pattern for p53 support a diagnosis of LGSC.[3]
- *LGSC versus EC*: This can be a problematic diagnosis on occasion; however, most LGSCs show dominant papillary architecture not seen

in EC. WT1 immunostaining, positive in LGSC but not EC, can be used in problematic cases.

- *EC versus MC*: The presence of a borderline or benign mucinous component in most MCs will serve to establish a diagnosis of MC, with ER immunostaining (strong and diffusely positive in most EC, and typically negative or weak/focal in MC) reserved for occasional challenging cases.
- *Primary ovarian carcinoma versus metastasis*: There is now awareness of the ability of metastases from extragenital (vermiform appendix, colon, pancreas, stomach) or genital (endocervix, endometrium) primary sites to involve the ovary and present with an ovarian mass and this has led to improved recognition of these metastatic carcinomas.[1]
- *Ovarian carcinomas of mixed histotype*: Although diagnosis of mixed carcinoma was commonly made in the past, this category has been removed from the 2014 WHO classification, as it has become clear that entities such as mixed serous and CCC or mixed serous and EC, are vanishingly rare, and that more than 99% of ovarian carcinomas will be of a single histotype, with the most common mixed carcinomas being those associated with endometriosis, for example, mixed clear cell and endometrioid carcinoma.[58]

HEREDITARY BREAST AND OVARIAN CANCER SYNDROME

HBOC syndrome is the most common cause of inherited breast and ovarian cancer[59,60] (**Box 1**).

It accounts for a large majority of those cases of ovarian cancer in which inherited susceptibility is a factor.[60] Henry Lynch and colleagues were the first to provide evidence of an autosomal dominant syndrome associated with increased risk of both breast and ovarian cancer in the 1970s. In 1990, the syndrome was further characterized, as the first gene associated with the syndrome (*BRCA1*, BReast CAncer) located on 17q21was identified.[61] A second gene (*BRCA2*), located at chromosome 13q12.3, was identified a year later.[59] These 2 genes account for more than 95% of cases of HBOC syndrome; a number of other genes were subsequently identified as being associated with rare cases of HBOC syndrome, including *RAD51*, *CHEK2*, and other genes.[62] The association of HBOC syndrome with early-onset breast cancer was noted and the initial focus within the scientific community was on breast cancer at the expense of other types of cancers associated with this syndrome, including gynecologic cancers. However, within the past decade, there has been growing recognition of the role *BRCA1* and *BRCA2* mutations play in development of ovarian cancer.

Although they have other functions, *BRCA1* and *BRCA2* (as well as the other genes less frequently mutated in HBOC syndrome, including *RAD51*) are critical for repair of double-stranded DNA breaks through homologous recombination. The BRCA1 and BRCA2 proteins combine with other proteins to form the BRCA-associated genome surveillance complex (BASC).[60] The BASC then identifies errors in double-stranded DNA using the homologous sister chromatid as the template to effect

---

Box 1
Hereditary breast and ovarian cancer (HBOC) syndrome

- Autosomal dominant cancer syndrome that is the most common cause of hereditary ovarian cancer
- *BRCA* 1 and *BRCA2* account for 95% of cases
- Other genes, including RAD51 and CHEK2, account for remaining cases
- *BRCA1* and *BRCA2* are critical for repair of double-stranded DNA breaks
- Ovarian tumors associated with HBOC syndrome are virtually all high-grade serous carcinoma (HGSC)
- Women with HBOC syndrome have an estimated 45% lifetime risk of developing HGSC
- No defining morphologic or immunohistochemical features associated with HGSC in these patients, compared with sporadic HGSC
- Risk-reducing surgery (bilateral salpingo-oophorectomy at age 40 or 5 years before earliest presentation of HGSC within kindred) has reduced the risk of developing HGSC by 98%
- Referral of patients newly diagnosed with tubo-ovarian HGSC will identify patients with unsuspected HBOC syndrome, and facilitate identifying affected family members who stand to benefit from risk-reducing surgery

high-fidelity repair. The alternative mechanism of repair of double-strand breaks is nonhomologous end joining (NHEJ).

Women with HBOC syndrome have an estimated 45% lifetime risk of developing HGSC. The risk for developing ovarian cancer by age 70 is 35% to 45% for *BRCA1* mutation carriers and 13% to 23% for *BRCA2* mutation carriers.[60] Although patients with HBOC develop ovarian cancer at a slightly earlier age, on average, than patients with nonhereditary ovarian cancer, the difference is small and is not useful in identifying patients with the syndrome.

The literature on the histologic features of ovarian cancer developing in patients with HBOC syndrome is confusing, and can best be understood if those studies are divided into those in which there has been no central pathology review, with application of modern diagnostic criteria, and studies in which such central review has taken place. The multicenter CIMBA study, published recently, on more than 1000 ovarian cancers arising in patients with known germline *BRCA1* or *BRCA2* mutations,[63] is the best example of the former type of study. These have shown convincingly that the ovarian cancers associated with HBOC syndrome are nonmucinous carcinomas, and not borderline tumors or nonepithelial tumors, but the histotype of the carcinomas has varied from study to study. In contrast, studies with central pathology review have shown that virtually all ovarian tumors associated with HBOC syndrome are HGSC.[64,65] Occasional cases of non-HGSC arising in patients with HBOC syndrome have been reported, but too few to establish whether they were associated with the syndrome/underlying genetic abnormality, or seen by chance alone in a patient with the syndrome. Although the breast cancers associated with *BRCA1* mutations show very significant differences compared with sporadic cases (ie, more likely to be of basal-like type), no such differences have been noted between the *BRCA1* and *BRCA2* associated and sporadic HGSCs. There are no defining morphologic or immunohistochemical features associated with HGSC in patients with HBOC syndrome, compared with sporadic cases, although weak associations have been noted with SET (Solid, pseudoEndometrioid, and Transitional) morphology,[66] missense p53 mutations, and the presence of tumor-infiltrating lymphocytes.[65] It is important to note that HBOC syndrome is not associated with serous carcinomas of the endometrium.[67]

Initial management of HGSC in patients with HBOC syndrome is identical to that of sporadic HGSC, and most syndromic HGSCs are platinum sensitive. Although the prognosis in the first years is better for patients with HGSC associated with HBOC syndrome, by 5 years this difference in prognosis has disappeared.[68] Therapy targeted against the defect in homologous recombination in HGSC (both hereditary and sporadic) has emerged, as inhibiters of PARP kill tumor cells through inhibition of a second DNA repair pathway, leading to apoptosis.[69] Patients known to have HBOC syndrome are offered risk-reducing surgery, consisting of bilateral salpingo-oophorectomy at age 40, or 5 years before the earliest presentation of HGSC within the kindred. This is remarkably effective in preventing the development of HGSC (approximately 98% reduction) and also halves breast cancer risk.[70]

As pathologists have improved their ability to recognize and diagnose the ovarian epithelial cancer histotypes accurately, we are able to aid in the identification of women who may be affected by HBOC syndrome. We recommend that all women with a diagnosis of HGSC be referred for genetic counseling, as 15% to 25% of women who develop HGSC will have HBOC syndrome.[71] If they are found to have a mutation in one of the genes associated with HBOC syndrome, testing can be offered to relatives, with risk-reducing surgery offered to those found to have HBOC syndrome. The significance of this diagnosis of HBOC for the family members of these women presenting with HGSC cannot be overstated.

LYNCH SYNDROME (HEREDITARY NONPOLYPOSIS COLORECTAL CANCER SYNDROME)

LS is an autosomal dominant cancer syndrome associated with increased risk of developing colonic, endometrial, ovarian, upper gastrointestinal, pancreatic, and ureteric cancer (Box 2). In the literature, the focus of LS has been predominantly on colorectal carcinoma but recently, there has been growing recognition of the role LS plays in development of gynecologic malignancies. LS was first reported by Dr Henry Lynch in the 1970s when he observed clustering of cancers within families in his practice.[59] Approximately 1 of 300 (1 of 1000–1 of 200) individuals within the general population are affected by LS. The lifetime risk of developing ovarian cancers in women with LS is 8% as compared with 1.4% for the general population.[72,73] Age of onset of ovarian cancer in the general population is approximately 60 years versus 42 to 49 years in LS.[74] Approximately 50% of the sentinel cases of LS are diagnosed based on endometrial or ovarian cancer.[75] Most ovarian cancers in LS are stage I or II.[74]

> **Box 2**
> **Lynch syndrome (LS)**
>
> - Autosomal dominant cancer syndrome associated with increased risk of developing colonic, endometrial, ovarian, upper gastrointestinal, pancreatic, and ureteric cancer
> - Lifetime risk of developing ovarian cancers in women with LS is 8%
> - Caused by defects in DNA mismatch repair (MMR)
> - Four most commonly mutated MMR proteins are MSH2, MSH6, PMS2, and MLH1
> - Mismatch repair proteins may be inactivated as a result of germline mutation or through a somatic (nonheritable) event such as promoter hypermethylation
> - Age of onset of ovarian cancer is younger in LS than in the general population (60 years vs 42–49 years)
> - 50% of the sentinel cases of LS in women are endometrial or ovarian cancers
> - LS is associated with 2 histotypes of ovarian cancer: endometrioid and clear cell
> - Although mixed carcinomas are rare, 20% of LS cases are associated with mixed endometrioid and clear cell histotypes
> - Reflex testing of newly diagnosed endometrial carcinomas and endometrioid or clear cell ovarian carcinomas can identify LS, and allow these patients and affected family members to be offered appropriate surveillance and risk-reducing surgery

LS is caused by defects in the DNA mismatch repair (MMR) mechanism, provided by a family of enzymes, including mutL homolog 1 (MLH1), mutS homolog 2 (MSH2), mutS homolog 3 (MSH3), mutS homolog 6 (MSH6), postmeiotic segregation increased 1 (PMS1), and postmeiotic segregation increased 2 (PMS2).[76] Patients with LS are born with a mutation in one allele and develop a somatic mutation in the intact allele later on in life.[74] For patients with endometrioid, clear cell, or undifferentiated ovarian carcinomas, however, the likelihood of LS is similar to that of patients with endometrial or colorectal carcinoma, and thus reflex MMR testing is recommended for these ovarian carcinoma histotypes[77,78] (Fig. 2). These histotypes of ovarian carcinoma are also strongly associated with endometriosis and are thought to arise from endometrial glandular epithelial cells; that is, the same cell type as EC arising within the uterus.[79]

Histologically, lymphocyte infiltrates are not a common finding within LS-associated ovarian epithelial cancers. Two studies report no association with tumor infiltrating lymphocytes (TILs),

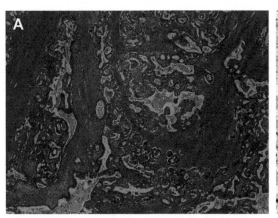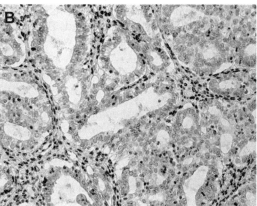

Fig. 2. (*A*) EC of the ovary is one of the histotypes (along with CCC) associated with LS. Note the well-formed glandular spaces typical of EC, whether arising in the endometrium or from endometriosis (H&E, 40×). (*B*) Isolated loss of expression of MSH6, although not diagnostic of LS, is associated with a high likelihood of an underlying mutation in the *MSH6* gene (MSH6, 200×).

peritumoral lymphocytes, or dedifferentiated morphology.[78,80] Of interest, mixed carcinomas account for 20% of the LS cohort, raising the possibility that intratumoral heterogeneity may be a morphologic feature of LS–ovarian carcinoma.[78] This finding is not surprising given that extensive sampling of MSI-H (microsatellite instability-high) colorectal cancers demonstrated widespread intratumoral heterogeneity with areas of the tumor showing TGFRBII mutations with poorly differentiated morphology.[81]

LS can be detected with reflex molecular testing in patients presenting with an LS-associated malignancy by looking for a loss of 1 of the 4 commonly mutated mismatch repair proteins (MSH2, MSH6, PMS2, or MLH1) within ovarian carcinomas of either endometrioid or clear cell type.[78] A loss of MSH2, MSH6, or PMS2 is strongly associated with LS, whereas a loss of MLH1 is often associated with inactivation by hypermethylation as a somatic event. Testing of MLH1 and MSH2 together will identify 90% to 95% of the germline mutations. When MSH6 and PMS2 are added, an additional 3% to 10% can be detected.[74] If all 4 proteins are expressed, then there is a normal phenotype. If one of the proteins is absent, then there is an abnormal phenotype. Care has to be taken when interpreting these stains. If MMR is not expressed in the background noncarcinoma tissue, then the abnormal study is not valid, as the internal control should show intact MMR expression. Because MLH1 is linked to PMS2 and MSH2 is linked to MSH6, then a negative MLH1 or MSH2 will result in PMS2 and MSH6 not being able to be interpreted by immunohistochemistry.

Other limitations of MMR staining include loss of expression in the absence of a germline mutation. Any of the 4 common MMR genes listed previously may be inactivated by promotor hypermethylation without mutations. As patients age, their DNA becomes methylated. Therefore, false-positive results will increase with the age of the patients.[82]

SUMMARY

The 2 common autosomal dominant cancer susceptibility syndromes, HBOC syndrome and LS, are both associated with an increased risk of developing ovarian carcinoma. The patients with HBOC have a lifetime risk of up to 50% for development of high-grade serous carcinoma of tube or ovary, whereas patients with LS have an approximately 10% lifetime risk of developing EC or CCC of the ovary. Testing all patients presenting with tubo-ovarian high-grade serous carcinoma for mutations associated with HBOC syndrome,

and screening all patients presenting with EC or CCC of the ovary for loss of expression of MMR proteins can identify patients with undiagnosed underlying hereditary cancer susceptibility syndromes and allow early diagnosis of these syndromes in relatives, so that appropriate surveillance and/or risk-reducing surgery can be offered.

REFERENCES

1. Kurman RJ, Carcangiu ML, Herrington CS, et al. WHO classification of tumours of female reproductive organs. 4th edition. Lyon (France): International Agency for Research on Cancer (IARC); 2014. p. 307.
2. Köbel M, Kalloger SE, Baker PM, et al. Diagnosis of ovarian carcinoma cell type is highly reproducible: a transcanadian study. Am J Surg Pathol 2010;34(7): 984–93.
3. Köbel M, Bak J, Bertelsen BII, et al. Ovarian carcinoma histotype determination is highly reproducible, and is improved through the use of immunohistochemistry. Histopathology 2014;64(7):1004–13.
4. Ferlay J, Shin H-RR, Bray F, et al. Estimates of worldwide burden of cancer in 2008: GLOBOCAN 2008. Int J Cancer 2010;127(12):2893–917.
5. Malpica A, Deavers M, Tornos C, et al. Interobserver and intraobserver variability of a two-tier system for grading ovarian serous carcinoma. Am J Surg Pathol 2007;31(8):1168.
6. Cancer Genome Atlas Research Network. Integrated genomic analyses of ovarian carcinoma. Nature 2011;474(7353):609–15.
7. Bashashati A, Ha G, Tone A, et al. Distinct evolutionary trajectories of primary high-grade serous ovarian cancers revealed through spatial mutational profiling. J Pathol 2013;231(1):21–34.
8. Köbel M, Reuss A, Bois A, et al. The biological and clinical value of p53 expression in pelvic high-grade serous carcinomas. J Pathol 2010;222(2): 191–8.
9. Singh N, Gilks CB, Wilkinson N, et al. The secondary Müllerian system, field effect, BRCA, and tubal fimbria: our evolving understanding of the origin of tubo-ovarian high-grade serous carcinoma and why assignment of primary site matters. Pathology 2015;47(5):423–31.
10. Auersperg N, Wong AS, Choi KC, et al. Ovarian surface epithelium: biology, endocrinology, and pathology. Endocr Rev 2001;22(2):255–88.
11. Feeley KM, Wells M. Precursor lesions of ovarian epithelial malignancy. Histopathology 2001;38(2): 87–95.
12. Gilks CB, Irving J, Köbel M, et al. Incidental nonuterine high-grade serous carcinomas arise in the fallopian tube in most cases: further evidence for the tubal origin of high-grade serous carcinomas. Am J Surg Pathol 2015;39(3):357–64.

13. Matsuno RK, Sherman ME, Visvanathan K, et al. Agreement for tumor grade of ovarian carcinoma: analysis of archival tissues from the surveillance, epidemiology, and end results residual tissue repository. Cancer Causes Control 2013;24(4):749–57.

14. Yemelyanova A, Mao T-LL, Nakayama N, et al. Low-grade serous carcinoma of the ovary displaying a macropapillary pattern of invasion. Am J Surg Pathol 2008;32(12):1800–6.

15. Vang R, Shih IeM, Kurman RJ. Ovarian low-grade and high-grade serous carcinoma: pathogenesis, clinicopathologic and molecular biologic features, and diagnostic problems. Adv Anat Pathol 2009; 16(5):267–82.

16. Bristow RE, Puri I, Chi DS. Cytoreductive surgery for recurrent ovarian cancer: a meta-analysis. Gynecol Oncol 2009;112(1):265–74.

17. Gershenson DM, Sun CC, Lu KH, et al. Clinical behavior of stage II-IV low-grade serous carcinoma of the ovary. Obstet Gynecol 2006;108(2):361–8.

18. Schmeler KM, Sun CC, Bodurka DC, et al. Neoadjuvant chemotherapy for low-grade serous carcinoma of the ovary or peritoneum. Gynecol Oncol 2008; 108(3):510–4.

19. Ali RH, Kalloger SE, Santos JL, et al. Stage II to IV low-grade serous carcinoma of the ovary is associated with a poor prognosis: a clinicopathologic study of 32 patients from a population-based tumor registry. Int J Gynecol Pathol 2013;32(6):529–35.

20. Köbel M, Kalloger SE, Huntsman DG, et al. Differences in tumor type in low-stage versus high-stage ovarian carcinomas. Int J Gynecol Pathol 2010; 29(3):203–11.

21. Fukunaga M, Nomura K, Ishikawa E, et al. Ovarian atypical endometriosis: its close association with malignant epithelial tumours. Histopathology 1997; 30(3):249–55.

22. Ogawa S, Kaku T, Amada S, et al. Ovarian endometriosis associated with ovarian carcinoma: a clinicopathological and immunohistochemical study. Gynecol Oncol 2000;77(2):298–304.

23. Jones S, Wang T-LL, Shih IeM, et al. Frequent mutations of chromatin remodeling gene ARID1A in ovarian clear cell carcinoma. Science 2010; 330(6001):228–31.

24. Wiegand KC, Shah SP, Al-Agha OM, et al. ARID1A mutations in endometriosis-associated ovarian carcinomas. N Engl J Med 2010; 363(16):1532–43.

25. Campbell IG, Russell SE, Choong DY, et al. Mutation of the PIK3CA gene in ovarian and breast cancer. Cancer Res 2004;64(21):7678–81.

26. Kuo K-TT, Mao T-LL, Jones S, et al. Frequent activating mutations of PIK3CA in ovarian clear cell carcinoma. Am J Pathol 2009;174(5):1597–601.

27. Yamamoto S, Tsuda H, Takano M, et al. PIK3CA mutation is an early event in the development of endometriosis-associated ovarian clear cell adenocarcinoma. J Pathol 2011;225(2):189–94.

28. Sato N, Tsunoda H, Nishida M, et al. Loss of heterozygosity on 10q23.3 and mutation of the tumor suppressor gene PTEN in benign endometrial cyst of the ovary: possible sequence progression from benign endometrial cyst to endometrioid carcinoma and clear cell carcinoma of the ovary. Cancer Res 2000;60(24):7052–6.

29. Lu F-II, Gilks CB, Mulligan A-MM, et al. Prevalence of loss of expression of DNA mismatch repair proteins in primary epithelial ovarian tumors. Int J Gynecol Pathol 2012;31(6):524–31.

30. Cai KQ, Albarracin C, Rosen D, et al. Microsatellite instability and alteration of the expression of hMLH1 and hMSH2 in ovarian clear cell carcinoma. Hum Pathol 2004;35(5):552–9.

31. Jensen KC, Mariappan MR, Putcha GV, et al. Microsatellite instability and mismatch repair protein defects in ovarian epithelial neoplasms in patients 50 years of age and younger. Am J Surg Pathol 2008; 32(7):1029–37.

32. Anglesio MS, Carey MS, Köbel M, et al. Clear cell carcinoma of the ovary: a report from the first Ovarian Clear Cell Symposium, June 24th, 2010. Gynecol Oncol 2011;121(2):407–15.

33. Chan JK, Teoh D, Hu JM, et al. Do clear cell ovarian carcinomas have poorer prognosis compared to other epithelial cell types? A study of 1411 clear cell ovarian cancers. Gynecol Oncol 2008;109(3):370–6.

34. Sugiyama T, Kamura T, Kigawa J, et al. Clinical characteristics of clear cell carcinoma of the ovary: a distinct histologic type with poor prognosis and resistance to platinum-based chemotherapy. Cancer 2000;88(11):2584–9.

35. DePriest PD, Banks ER, Powell DE, et al. Endometrioid carcinoma of the ovary and endometriosis: the association in postmenopausal women. Gynecol Oncol 1992;47(1):71–5.

36. Mostoufizadeh M, Scully RE. Malignant tumors arising in endometriosis. Clin Obstet Gynecol 1980;23(3):951–63.

37. Storey DJ, Rush R, Stewart M, et al. Endometrioid epithelial ovarian cancer: 20 years of prospectively collected data from a single center. Cancer 2008; 112(10):2211–20.

38. Irving JA, Catasús L, Gallardo A, et al. Synchronous endometrioid carcinomas of the uterine corpus and ovary: alterations in the beta-catenin (CTNNB1) pathway are associated with independent primary tumors and favorable prognosis. Hum Pathol 2005; 36(6):605–19.

39. Kline RC, Wharton JT, Atkinson EN, et al. Endometrioid carcinoma of the ovary: retrospective review of 145 cases. Gynecol Oncol 1990;39(3):337–46.

40. Zaino RJ, Unger ER, Whitney C. Synchronous carcinomas of the uterine corpus and ovary. Gynecol Oncol 1984;19(3):329–35.

41. Catasús L, Bussaglia E, Rodrguez I, et al. Molecular genetic alterations in endometrioid carcinomas of the ovary: similar frequency of beta-catenin abnormalities but lower rate of microsatellite instability and PTEN alterations than in uterine endometrioid carcinomas. Hum Pathol 2004;35(11):1360–8.

42. Obata K, Morland SJ, Watson RH, et al. Frequent PTEN/MMAC mutations in endometrioid but not serous or mucinous epithelial ovarian tumors. Cancer Res 1998;58(10):2095–7.

43. Wu R, Zhai Y, Fearon ER, et al. Diverse mechanisms of beta-catenin deregulation in ovarian endometrioid adenocarcinomas. Cancer Res 2001;61(22):8247–55.

44. Wright K, Wilson P, Morland S, et al. Beta-catenin mutation and expression analysis in ovarian cancer: exon 3 mutations and nuclear translocation in 16% of endometrioid tumours. Int J Cancer 1999;82(5):625–9.

45. Sagae S, Kobayashi K, Nishioka Y, et al. Mutational analysis of beta-catenin gene in Japanese ovarian carcinomas: frequent mutations in endometrioid carcinomas. Jpn J Cancer Res 1999;90(5):510–5.

46. Moreno-Bueno G, Gamallo C, Pérez-Gallego L, et al. beta-Catenin expression pattern, beta-catenin gene mutations, and microsatellite instability in endometrioid ovarian carcinomas and synchronous endometrial carcinomas. Diagn Mol Pathol 2001;10(2):116–22.

47. Zaino RJ, Brady MF, Lele SM, et al. Advanced stage mucinous adenocarcinoma of the ovary is both rare and highly lethal: a Gynecologic Oncology Group study. Cancer 2011;117(3):554–62.

48. Schiavone MB, Herzog TJ, Lewin SN, et al. Natural history and outcome of mucinous carcinoma of the ovary. Am J Obstet Gynecol 2011;205(5):480.e1–8.

49. Kerr SE, Flotte AB, McFalls MJ, et al. Matching maternal isodisomy in mucinous carcinomas and associated ovarian teratomas provides evidence of germ cell derivation for some mucinous ovarian tumors. Am J Surg Pathol 2013;37(8):1229–35.

50. Garrett AP, Lee KR, Colitti CR, et al. K-ras mutation may be an early event in mucinous ovarian tumorigenesis. Int J Gynecol Pathol 2001;20(3):244–51.

51. Cuatrecasas M, Villanueva A, Matias-Guiu X, et al. K-ras mutations in mucinous ovarian tumors: a clinicopathologic and molecular study of 95 cases. Cancer 1997;79(8):1581–6.

52. Ichikawa Y, Nishida M, Suzuki H, et al. Mutation of K-ras protooncogene is associated with histological subtypes in human mucinous ovarian tumors. Cancer Res 1994;54(1):33–5.

53. Mok SC, Bell DA, Knapp RC, et al. Mutation of K-ras protooncogene in human ovarian epithelial tumors of borderline malignancy. Cancer Res 1993;53(7):1489–92.

54. Anglesio MS, Kommoss S, Tolcher MC, et al. Molecular characterization of mucinous ovarian tumours supports a stratified treatment approach with HER2 targeting in 19% of carcinomas. J Pathol 2013;229(1):111–20.

55. Schwartz DR, Kardia SL, Shedden KA, et al. Gene expression in ovarian cancer reflects both morphology and biological behavior, distinguishing clear cell from other poor-prognosis ovarian carcinomas. Cancer Res 2002;62(16):4722–9.

56. Wu R, Hendrix-Lucas N, Kuick R, et al. Mouse model of human ovarian endometrioid adenocarcinoma based on somatic defects in the Wnt/beta-catenin and PI3K/Pten signaling pathways. Cancer Cell 2007;11(4):321–33.

57. DeLair D, Oliva E, Köbel M, et al. Morphologic spectrum of immunohistochemically characterized clear cell carcinoma of the ovary: a study of 155 cases. Am J Surg Pathol 2011;35(1):36–44.

58. Mackenzie R, Talhouk A, Eshragh S, et al. Morphologic and molecular characteristics of mixed epithelial ovarian cancers. Am J Surg Pathol 2015;39(11):1548–57.

59. Lynch HT, Snyder C, Casey MJ. Hereditary ovarian and breast cancer: what have we learned? Ann Oncol 2013;24(Suppl 8):viii83–95.

60. Girolimetti G, Perrone AM, Santini D, et al. BRCA-associated ovarian cancer: from molecular genetics to risk management. Biomed Res Int 2014;2014:787143.

61. Hall JM, Lee MK, Newman B, et al. Linkage of early-onset familial breast cancer to chromosome 17q21. Science 1990;250(4988):1684–9.

62. Walsh T, Casadei S, Lee MK, et al. Mutations in 12 genes for inherited ovarian, fallopian tube, and peritoneal carcinoma identified by massively parallel sequencing. Proc Natl Acad Sci U S A 2011;108(44):18032–7.

63. Mavaddat N, Barrowdale D, Andrulis IL, et al. Pathology of breast and ovarian cancers among BRCA1 and BRCA2 mutation carriers: results from the Consortium of Investigators of Modifiers of BRCA1/2 (CIMBA). Cancer Epidemiol Biomarkers Prev 2012;21(1):134–47.

64. Risch HA, McLaughlin JR, Cole DE, et al. Prevalence and penetrance of germline BRCA1 and BRCA2 mutations in a population series of 649 women with ovarian cancer. Am J Hum Genet 2001;68(3):700–10.

65. McAlpine JN, Porter H, Köbel M, et al. BRCA1 and BRCA2 mutations correlate with TP53 abnormalities and presence of immune cell infiltrates in ovarian

high-grade serous carcinoma. Mod Pathol 2012; 25(5):740–50.

66. Hussein YR, Ducie JA, Arnold AG, et al. Invasion patterns of metastatic extrauterine high-grade serous carcinoma with BRCA germline mutation and correlation with clinical outcomes. Am J Surg Pathol 2015;40(3):404–9.

67. Kandoth C, Schultz N, Cherniack AD, et al. Integrated genomic characterization of endometrial carcinoma. Nature 2013;497(7447):67–73.

68. Candido-dos-Reis FJ, Song H, Goode EL, et al. Germline mutation in BRCA1 or BRCA2 and ten-year survival for women diagnosed with epithelial ovarian cancer. Clin Cancer Res 2015;21(3): 652–7.

69. Ricks TK, Chiu H-JJ, Ison G, et al. Successes and challenges of PARP inhibitors in cancer therapy. Front Oncol 2015;5:222.

70. Walker JL, Powell CB, Chen L-MM, et al. Society of Gynecologic Oncology recommendations for the prevention of ovarian cancer. Cancer 2015; 121(13):2108–20.

71. Schrader KA, Hurlburt J, Kalloger SE, et al. Germline BRCA1 and BRCA2 mutations in ovarian cancer: utility of a histology-based referral strategy. Obstet Gynecol 2012;120(2 Pt 1):235–40.

72. Aarnio M, Sankila R, Pukkala E, et al. Cancer risk in mutation carriers of DNA-mismatch-repair genes. Int J Cancer 1999;81(2):214–8.

73. Watson P, Vasen HF, Mecklin J-PP, et al. The risk of extra-colonic, extra-endometrial cancer in the Lynch syndrome. Int J Cancer 2008;123(2):444–9.

74. Nakamura K, Banno K, Yanokura M, et al. Features of ovarian cancer in Lynch syndrome (Review). Mol Clin Oncol 2014;2(6):909–16.

75. Lu KH, Dinh M, Kohlmann W, et al. Gynecologic cancer as a "sentinel cancer" for women with hereditary nonpolyposis colorectal cancer syndrome. Obstet Gynecol 2005;105(3):569–74.

76. Jascur T, Boland CR. Structure and function of the components of the human DNA mismatch repair system. Int J Cancer 2006;119(9):2030–5.

77. Chui MH, Gilks CB, Cooper K, et al. Identifying Lynch syndrome in patients with ovarian carcinoma: the significance of tumor subtype. Adv Anat Pathol 2013;20(6):378–86.

78. Chui MH, Ryan P, Radigan J, et al. The histomorphology of Lynch syndrome-associated ovarian carcinomas: toward a subtype-specific screening strategy. Am J Surg Pathol 2014;38(9):1173–81.

79. Lu Y, Cuellar-Partida G, Painter JN, et al. Shared genetics underlying epidemiological association between endometriosis and ovarian cancer. Hum Mol Genet 2015;24(20):5955–64.

80. Aysal A, Karnezis A, Medhi I, et al. Ovarian endometrioid adenocarcinoma: incidence and clinical significance of the morphologic and immunohistochemical markers of mismatch repair protein defects and tumor microsatellite instability. Am J Surg Pathol 2012;36(2):163–72.

81. Barnetson R, Jass J, Tse R, et al. Mutations associated with microsatellite unstable colorectal carcinomas exhibit widespread intratumoral heterogeneity. Genes Chromosomes Cancer 2000;29(2): 130–6.

82. Graham RP, Kerr SE, Butz ML, et al. Heterogenous MSH6 loss is a result of microsatellite instability within MSH6 and occurs in sporadic and hereditary colorectal and endometrial carcinomas. Am J Surg Pathol 2015;39(10):1370–6.

Lynch Syndrome
Female Genital Tract Cancer Diagnosis and Screening

Anne M. Mills, MD[a], Teri A. Longacre, MD[b],*

KEYWORDS

- Lynch syndrome • Hereditary nonpolyposis cancer syndrome • Mismatch repair proteins
- Microsatellite instability • Endometrial cancer • Ovarian cancer

ABSTRACT

Lynch syndrome is responsible for approximately 5% of endometrial cancers and 1% of ovarian cancers. The molecular basis for Lynch syndrome is a heritable functional deficiency in the DNA mismatch repair system, typically due to a germline mutation. This review discusses the rationales and relative merits of current Lynch syndrome screening tests for endometrial and ovarian cancers and provides pathologists with an informed algorithmic approach to Lynch syndrome testing in gynecologic cancers. Pitfalls in test interpretation and strategies to resolve discordant test results are presented. The potential role for next-generation sequencing panels in future screening efforts is discussed.

OVERVIEW

Lynch syndrome (LS), also known as Hereditary Nonpolyposis Colorectal Carcinoma (HNPCC) is an autosomal dominant cancer syndrome caused by inactivating germline mutations in the DNA mismatch repair (MMR) genes. The most frequent clinically relevant mutations occur in the *MLH1*, *MSH2*, *MSH6*, *PMS2*, and *EPCAM* genes. Patients with LS are at increased risk for multiple malignancies, including cancers of the colorectum, endometrium, ovary, stomach, urinary tract, hepatobiliary tract, small intestine, sebaceous gland, and brain.[1–3] Because LS has traditionally been approached as a colorectal carcinoma–dominated

syndrome, screening strategies have centered on colon cancer. However, women with LS are at equal, if not higher, risk for development of gynecologic malignancies when compared with their risk for colon cancer.[1] Moreover, more than half of affected patients present with a gynecologic malignancy, usually endometrial cancer, as their sentinel cancer.[4] The frequency of LS germline mutations in endometrial carcinomas has been estimated at 1.8% to 2.1%, which is similar to that in colon cancer.[5,6] However, recent literature indicates this may be closer to 5.9% in unselected patients with endometrial cancer.[5,7,8] Moreover, the lifetime risk for development of endometrial carcinoma in these patients (up to 60%) may exceed that for colorectal carcinoma.[1,2] For comparison, the current estimated lifetime risk for developing endometrial cancer in the general population is 2% to 3% for the average woman. LS accounts for approximately 2% of all ovarian cancers.[9] The reported lifetime risk of ovarian cancer in LS is 4% to 12%[1,3,9–16] Risk for ovarian cancer appears to be particularly high for patients with *MSH2* and *MSH6* mutations.[14,15] Patients with LS often present with ovarian tumors at relatively younger age (mean 40–48 years); unlike endometrial carcinoma in LS, most patients with ovarian cancer are younger than 50 years of age.[15,16]

Because a substantial number of women with LS first present with a gynecologic cancer, gynecologists and pathologists have the opportunity to identify women at potential risk for synchronous and metachronous tumors, particularly colon

Conflicts of Interest and Funding Statements: The authors have disclosed no significant relationships with or financial interest in any commercial companies pertaining to this article.

[a] Department of Pathology, University of Virginia, 1215 Lee Street, P.O. Box 800214, Charlottesville, VA 22908, USA; [b] Department of Pathology, Stanford University School of Medicine, Room L235, 300 Pasteur Drive, Stanford, CA 94305, USA

* Corresponding author.

E-mail address: longacre@stanford.edu

http://dx.doi.org/10.1016/j.path.2016.01.004
1875-9181/16/$ – see front matter © 2016 Elsevier Inc. All rights reserved.

cancer.[1,17] The time to development of a second cancer varies with a median time of 11 years for patients with endometrial cancer and 5.5 years for patients first diagnosed with ovarian cancer; timely detection of LS in these patients and their family members could lead to appropriate surveillance measures, and decreased morbidity and mortality from metachronous colon cancer.[4]

FUNCTION OF DNA MISMATCH REPAIR GENES

Mutations in the DNA-MMR genes involved in LS are typically associated with loss of function and high microsatellite instability (MSI-H).[18] Microsatellites are repetitive widely dispersed DNA sequences consisting of mono-, di-, or higher-order nucleotide repeats that are prone to replication errors due to inefficient binding of DNA polymerases. Normally these errors are corrected by the DNA-MMR system (DNA-MMR). Deficiencies in the DNA-MMR therefore results in MSI-H.[19] Microsatellite instability occurs as a result of genetic (MMR gene mutation) or epigenetic (most commonly, MLH1 promoter methylation) alterations.[20] Of the 20% to 25% of endometrial carcinomas that are MSI-H, 75% result from sporadic MLH1 promoter methylation. The minority are LS-associated tumors. Therefore, LS and MSI should not be used synonymously.

LYNCH SYNDROME FEMALE GENITAL TRACT TUMORS

LS endometrial cancers do not exhibit site-specific or morphology-specific features to the degree that is seen in LS colorectal cancer. Although it has been suggested that as many as one-third of tumors arising in the lower uterine segment may be LS, in reality it is probably more on the order of 10% to 15%.[21,22] The endometrial carcinomas can show a wide spectrum of histologic subtypes. Endometrioid carcinomas are the most common type, but nonendometrioid carcinomas, including serous carcinoma, clear cell carcinoma, and carcinosarcoma, are also observed in LS, often at comparatively younger ages than is typically associated with these tumors.[21,23,24] Several histologic features of uterine endometrioid cancers (eg, tumor-infiltrating lymphocytes, prominent peritumoral lymphocytes, tumor heterogeneity, undifferentiated or dedifferentiated histology) have been linked to microsatellite instability, but their predictive value in identifying a potential germline MMR protein mutation is less certain.[8,25–29]

One of the endometrial cancer subtypes that has been associated with microsatellite instability is undifferentiated endometrioid carcinoma (Fig. 1). Undifferentiated endometrial carcinoma is composed of solid, discohesive sheets of round or polygonal cells with vesicular nuclei and prominent nucleoli; no gland formation is present (see Fig. 1).[30] A myxoid matrix, rhabdoid cells, or lymphoepitheliomalike areas, defined as sheets of undifferentiated cells with a prominent lymphocytic infiltrate may be seen in undifferentiated endometrial carcinoma. When undifferentiated carcinoma is accompanied by a distinct component of well to moderately differentiated endometrioid carcinoma, it has been designated as dedifferentiated endometrial carcinoma.[31] Undifferentiated/dedifferentiated endometrial carcinomas are associated with MMR abnormalities and MSI-H.[32] Most are sporadic and associated with MLH1 promoter methylation.[23,25] Undifferentiated and dedifferentiated carcinomas appear to be particularly associated with abnormalities of MLH1/PMS2, both in the form of promoter methylation and germline mutations (see Fig. 1).[21]

> *Key Features*
> MORPHOLOGY
> OF MICROSATELLITE UNSTABLE
> ENDOMETRIOID ADENOCARCINOMA
>
> - Prominent peritumoral lymphocytes (apparent at scanning magnification)
> - Increased tumor-infiltrating lymphocytes (TILs); that is, lymphocytes located within the boundary of tumor cell nests or glands (TILs >42 per 10 high-power fields)
> - Tumor heterogeneity defined as 2 morphologically distinct tumor populations juxtaposed but not intimately admixed, each constituting at least 10% of the tumor volume
> - Undifferentiated or dedifferentiated histology

In contrast, the spectrum of ovarian tumors seen in LS differs from that of the general population. Most LS ovarian cancers are nonserous; most are endometrioid, clear cell, or undifferentiated carcinomas.[14,15] The endometrioid carcinomas are usually well to moderately differentiated, present at early stages, and appear to pursue a favorable clinical course.[12,15] Ovarian clear cell carcinoma, particularly in younger patients, is also strongly associated with LS; up to 14% to 17% of ovarian clear cell carcinomas are associated with MMR defects.[14,15] Approximately 10% of all ovarian carcinomas in patients 50 years of age or younger are associated with MMR defects, and most (60%) of these are clear cell carcinomas, with the remainder showing undifferentiated or endometrioid histology.[14]

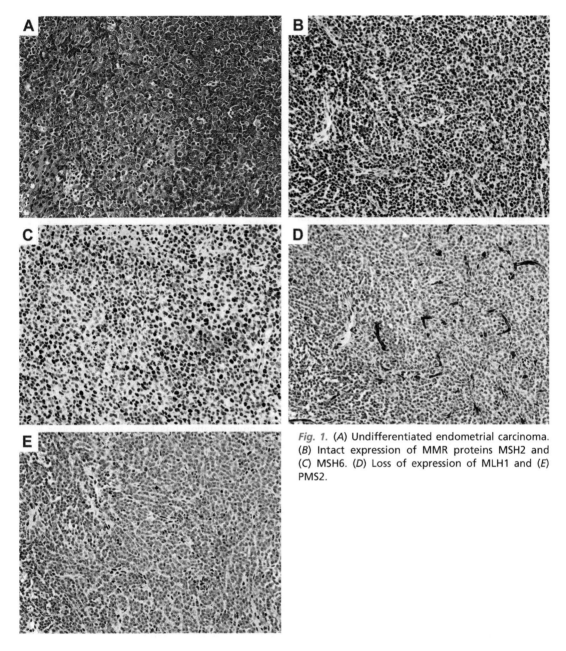

Fig. 1. (*A*) Undifferentiated endometrial carcinoma. (*B*) Intact expression of MMR proteins MSH2 and (*C*) MSH6. (*D*) Loss of expression of MLH1 and (*E*) PMS2.

Key Features
MORPHOLOGY OF MICROSATELLITE UNSTABLE OVARIAN CARCINOMAS

- Typically nonserous morphology
  - Endometrioid
  - Clear cell
  - Undifferentiated
- Synchronous endometrial primaries may be present

Some studies have reported an association between LS and presence of synchronous endometrioid carcinomas of the ovary and endometrium, but others have not found this association.[16,21] Synchronous uterine endometrioid carcinoma and ovarian clear cell carcinoma has been observed in women with mismatch protein repair defects, but the numbers of reported cases are few.[14,33]

There is no association between LS and endocervical adenocarcinoma.[34] Uterine and cervical mesenchymal tumors (leiomyosarcoma, endometrial stromal sarcoma, adenosarcoma) are also not currently considered to be LS tumors.[21]

LYNCH SYNDROME FEMALE GENITAL TRACT CANCER RISK DIFFERS BY MUTATIONAL STATUS

Endometrial cancer in women with LS is more frequently associated with *MSH2* and *MSH6* germline mutations than with germline mutations in *MLH1* and *PMS2*. In addition to these differences in prevalence, the penetrance of disease also differs among the mutated MMR genes. The current estimated cumulative endometrial cancer risk for women with *MLH1* or *MSH2* germline mutations ranges from 21% to 54% by age 70. In contrast, the current estimated lifetime risk for endometrial cancer for women with a germline mutation in *MSH6* is 16% to 71% by age 70, and the estimated lifetime risk for endometrial cancer for women with a germline mutation in *PMS2* is 12% by age 70.[35] The mean age of diagnosis of endometrial cancer is also higher (>50 years) in women with *MSH6* and *PMS2* germline mutations.

Although it is reported that most LS ovarian cancers are associated with *MLH1* or *MSH2* germline mutations, the data are insufficient to determine whether there are differences in penetrance. Most LS ovarian cancer appears to present in women younger than 50 years.

SCREENING FOR LYNCH SYNDROME

There are currently no uniform screening guidelines for detection of LS in patients who present with gynecologic cancers. Various screening modalities that use patient factors including age, personal history, and family history have been proposed and tested. The Amsterdam (**Box 1**) and Bethesda (**Box 2**) criteria focus primarily on colorectal carcinomas,[2,36,37] whereas the Society of Gynecologic Oncologists (SGO) guidelines focus on gynecologic tumors (**Box 3**).[38]

In general, LS should be a consideration in young patients with gynecologic cancers.[11] However, most women with LS present with endometrial cancer when they are older than 50 years, and this is particularly true for those with *MSH6* mutations.[5,11,21,39] Personal and/or family history of LS-associated tumors is extremely useful, but it is also not sufficiently sensitive. Up to 75% of patients with LS do not meet the Amsterdam criteria or Bethesda guidelines and do not have personal or family history suggestive of LS.[5,21] In one study, only 58% of endometrial carcinoma patients with LS met Amsterdam II criteria, whereas only 36% met revised Bethesda guidelines.[27]

Although some studies have advocated incorporation of tumor characteristics in the screening algorithm with some success, it is uncertain whether these screening programs are sufficiently sensitive in the detection of MMR abnormalities in patients with endometrial carcinoma.[25,27] A recent recommendation has been made to offer MMR deficiency testing to all patients newly diagnosed with endometrial cancer, irrespective of age and personal or family history.[21] This proposal is similar to that recently proposed for colorectal

---

Box 1
Amsterdam criteria for Lynch syndrome screening

Amsterdam Criteria I

- Three or more family members with a confirmed diagnosis of colorectal cancer, one of whom is a first-degree (parent, child, sibling) relative of the other two

- Two successive affected generations

- One or more colon cancers diagnosed in patients younger than age 50 years

- Familial adenomatous polyposis (FAP) has been excluded

Amsterdam Criteria II

- Three or more family members with hereditary nonpolyposis colorectal cancer (HNPCC)-related cancers, one of whom is a first-degree relative of the other two

- Two successive affected generations

- One or more of the HNPCC-related cancers diagnosed in patient younger than age 50 years

- FAP has been excluded

Data from Vasen HF, Watson P, Mecklin JP, et al. New clinical criteria for hereditary nonpolyposis colorectal cancer (HNPCC, Lynch syndrome) proposed by the International Collaborative group on HNPCC. Gastroenterology 1999;116:1453–6; and Vasen HF, Mecklin JP, Khan PM, et al. The international collaborative group on hereditary non-polyposis colorectal cancer (ICG-HNPCC). Dis Colon Rectum 1991;34:424–5.

Box 2
Revised Bethesda guidelines

- Diagnosed with colorectal cancer before the age of 50 years.

- Synchronous or metachronous colorectal or other Lynch syndrome (LS)/HNPCC-related tumors (which include stomach, bladder, ureter, renal pelvis, biliary tract, brain [glioblastoma], sebaceous gland adenomas, keratoacanthomas, and carcinoma of the small bowel), regardless of age.

- Colorectal cancer with a high microsatellite instability morphology that was diagnosed in a patient younger than 60 years.

- Colorectal cancer with one or more first-degree relatives with colorectal cancer or other LS/HNPCC-related tumors. One of the cancers must have been diagnosed before the age of 50 years (this includes adenoma, which must have been diagnosed before the age of 40 years).

- Colorectal cancer with 2 or more relatives with colorectal cancer or other LS/HNPCC-related tumors, regardless of age.

Data from Umar A, Boland CR, Terdiman JP, et al. Revised Bethesda guidelines for hereditary nonpolyposis colorectal cancer (Lynch syndrome) and microsatellite instability. J Natl Cancer Inst 2004;96:261–8.

---

cancer screening.[40,41] An alternative approach is universal screening for all women with endometrial cancer who are younger than 60 years.[8] Both screening procedures can be accomplished in a cost-effective model that incorporates the 2 MMR protein antibody panel.[42,43]

TESTING FOR LYNCH SYNDROME

GERMLINE MUTATIONAL ANALYSIS

Germline mutational analysis of the DNA MMR genes is the definitive test to establish a diagnosis of LS. However, mutation analysis is not an effective screening test, and should be used as a confirmatory test. Other tests including

immunohistochemistry (IHC), MSI analysis, *MLH1* methylation, and somatic mutation studies may serve as better screening tests.

IMMUNOHISTOCHEMISTRY FOR DNA MISMATCH REPAIR PROTEINS

IHC for DNA MMR proteins has been shown to be a sensitive and specific test for detection of MMR abnormalities in endometrial carcinoma.[44] When all 4 antibodies (MLH1, PMS2, MSH2, and MSH6) are used, IHC has a sensitivity of 91% and specificity of 83% for detecting MSI-high.[44] The lower specificity is likely due to mutations in *MSH6*, which can result in MSI-low or MS-stable tumors. In their functional state, the MMR proteins

---

Box 3
Society of Gynecologic Oncology (SGO) guidelines for referral for Lynch syndrome counseling

Patients with an increased likelihood of Lynch syndrome and for whom genetic assessment is recommended

- Patients with endometrial or colorectal cancer with evidence of microsatellite instability or loss of DNA mismatch repair protein (MLH1, MSH2, MSH6, PMS2) on immunohistochemistry.

- Patients with a first-degree or second-degree relative with a known mutation in a mismatch repair gene.

- Families with few female relatives, as this may lead to an underrepresentation of female cancers despite the presence of a predisposing family mutation.

- Hysterectomy and/or oophorectomy at a young age in multiple family members, as this might mask a hereditary gynecologic cancer predisposition.

- Presence of adoption in the lineage.

Data from Lancaster JM, Powell CB, Chen LM, et al. Society of Gynecologic Oncology statement on risk assessment for inherited gynecologic cancer predispositions. Gynecol Oncol 2015;136:3–7.

form dimers: MLH1 dimerizes with PMS2 and MSH2 dimerizes with MSH6. MLH1 and MSH2 are the obligatory partners in these dimers; mutations in MLH1 and MSH2 lead to concurrent loss of PMS2 and MSH6, respectively (Table 1). Therefore *MLH1* promoter methylation or mutation will result in IHC loss of both MLH1 and PMS2 (Fig. 2). Similarly, mutations in *MSH2* will lead to IHC loss of both MSH2 and MSH6. However, isolated loss of PMS2 (Fig. 3) and MSH6 (Fig. 4) can occur due to *PMS2* and *MSH6* mutations, respectively. Because loss of MLH1 and PMS2 may be due to *MLH1* promoter methylation or germline mutation in *MLH1*, further testing is required to differentiate between genetic versus epigenetic mechanisms of loss. Until recently, loss of MSH2 and/or MSH6 was considered to be virtually diagnostic of LS; however, the discovery of somatic mutations involving these MMR genes has contributed another layer of complexity to LS testing.[45–47]

Loss of more than 2 proteins or loss of MMR proteins in other combinations is rare and occurs when epigenetic methylation develops in association with a germline mutation.[48] Recent data suggest that a 2-antibody panel (composed of PMS2 and MSH6) is as effective as the 4-antibody panel for detection of MMR abnormalities.[42,43]

IHC has numerous advantages as a screening test. It is simple, easily available, and relatively inexpensive (up to threefold less expensive than MSI testing). Another advantage of IHC is that it can help direct gene sequencing to 1 or 2 specific genes, based on the pattern of loss. This algorithm of IHC followed by directed gene sequencing has been shown to be the most cost-effective strategy for detection of LS in patients with endometrial cancer.[49] IHC is particularly advantageous in tumors with *MSH6* mutations, as these can be MSI-low or MSI-stable and may therefore be missed by MSI analysis alone.

The interpretation of IHC for MMR proteins can sometimes be difficult. Intact expression is indicated by the presence of nuclear staining; nuclear membrane, nucleolar, and cytoplasmic staining should not be interpreted as intact expression. There should be complete loss of staining in all tumor cells for an interpretation of IHC loss of a protein. Care should be taken to examine for presence of internal positive control (stroma, lymphocytes, or normal endometrium), which should show nuclear staining. Nuclear staining of tumor cells, even when focal and weak, should be interpreted as retained staining. MSH2 and PMS2 stains are usually straightforward and easy to interpret. However, MSH6 and MLH1 stains can be challenging. MSH6 expression can be heterogeneous with some areas appearing to lack expression, whereas others clearly demonstrate nuclear expression; hence small biopsies (eg, tissue microarrays in research or small biopsies in clinical practice) may be insufficient to evaluate MSH6 protein deficiency. If it continues to be problematic, the stain should be interpreted as equivocal or inconclusive, and alternative testing mechanisms should be pursued. Because many of these tumors harbor numerous intraepithelial lymphocytes, it may be difficult in some cases to distinguish nuclear expression in the infiltrating lymphocytes from that of the tumor cell nuclei, thus resulting in a false-negative test (ie, the tumor is interpreted as MMR proficient, when in fact it is MMR deficient). IHC does not recognize all germline mutations, as occasional mutations result in loss of function but expression is preserved.[5]

MICROSATELLITE INSTABILITY ANALYSIS

MSI analysis by polymerase chain reaction uses dinucleotide and mononucleotide markers. DNA from tumor and normal tissue (or plasma) is isolated and tested with a panel of 5 microsatellite markers. The microsatellite markers from the tumor and normal DNA are then compared to detect somatic alterations. The most commonly used panel incorporates the 5 mononucleotide and dinucleotide microsatellite markers recommended by the National Cancer Institute (NCI): BAT25, BAT26, D2S123, D5S346, and D17S250.[50] However, a panel of 5 mononucleotide markers (BAT25, BAT26, NR21, NR24, and NR27) has been shown to be as effective and reproducible as the NCI panel, with superior performance.[51] When a tumor shows MSI at 2 or more loci, it is considered MSI-high, instability at 1 locus is

Table 1	
Common patterns of mismatch repair protein loss	
MMR IHC Loss Pattern	**Implication**
MLH1/PMS2	Epigenetic *MLH1* promoter methylation or possible *MLH1* mutation
PMS2	Possible *PMS2* mutation or possible *MLH1* mutation
MSH2/MHS6	Possible *MSH2* or *EPCAM* mutation
MSH6	Possible *MSH6* mutation

Abbreviations: IHC, immunohistochemistry; MMR, mismatch repair.

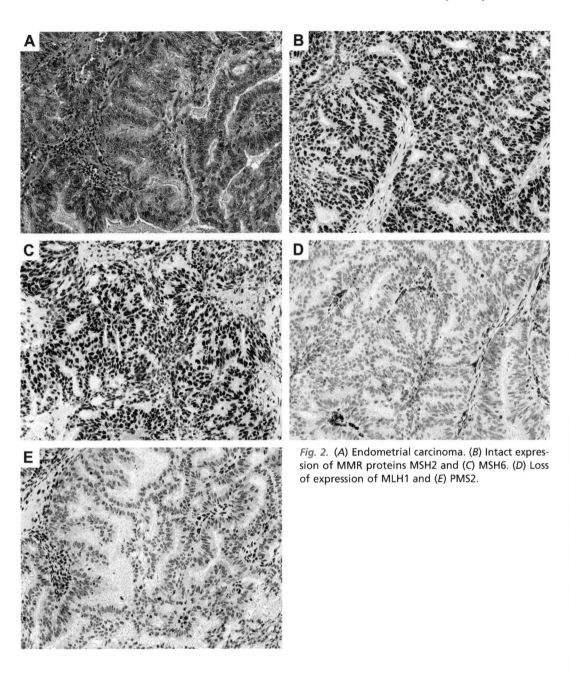

Fig. 2. (A) Endometrial carcinoma. (B) Intact expression of MMR proteins MSH2 and (C) MSH6. (D) Loss of expression of MLH1 and (E) PMS2.

interpreted as MSI-low and if no instability is detected, it is considered MS-stable. The disadvantages of MSI analysis compared with IHC are that it is more expensive and requires a molecular laboratory; normal DNA is required. Also, it may not detect carcinomas associated with *MSH6* mutations, which may be MSI-low or stable. MSI can result from *MLH1* promoter methylation or germline mutations, and this test cannot differentiate between these 2 mechanisms. A recent study evaluating the efficacy of MMR IHC versus MSI

in the evaluation of endometrial cancer demonstrated a 93% concordance between the 2 testing methodologies.[52]

MLH1 PROMOTER METHYLATION ASSAY

This test detects the presence of *MLH1* promoter methylation, which is an acquired phenomenon that results in inactivation of *MLH1* with resultant loss of MLH1 protein by IHC. If a tumor shows *MLH1* promoter methylation, it is

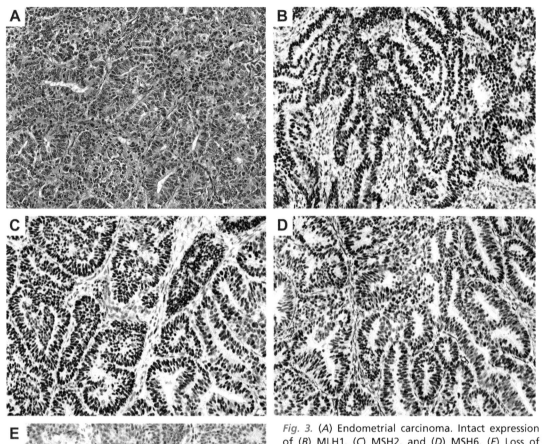

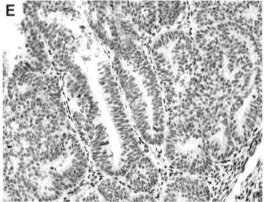

Fig. 3. (A) Endometrial carcinoma. Intact expression of (B) MLH1, (C) MSH2, and (D) MSH6. (E) Loss of PMS2 expression.

unlikely to be LS associated. In contrast, a tumor that shows loss of MLH1 and PMS2 by IHC but no evidence of promoter methylation is highly likely to be associated with LS. Because sporadic colorectal carcinomas with *MLH1* promoter methylation frequently show *BRAF* mutations, assessment for *BRAF* mutation is an effective and relatively inexpensive test for possible *MLH1* promoter methylation in colorectal cancer.[53] However, methylation analysis is required for MLH1-deficient endometrial carcinomas, as

BRAF mutations have not been detected in these tumors.[21,54] *MLH1* methylation testing on tumor tissue alone will not distinguish LS cases with a constitutional *MLH1* epimutation.

DNA MISMATCH REPAIR GENE MUTATION ANALYSIS

This is a confirmatory test to establish a diagnosis of LS and is generally only performed if 1 or more of the previously described screening tests

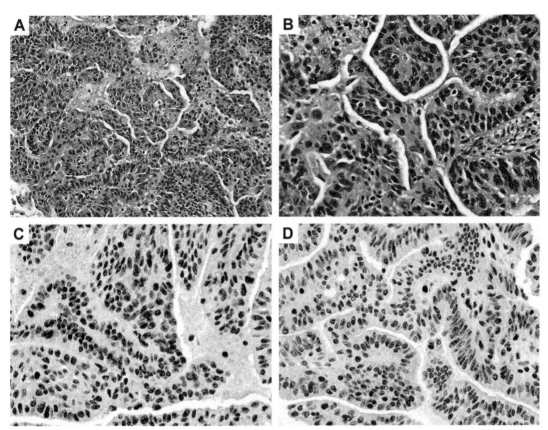

Fig. 4. (*A, B*) Endometrial carcinoma. (*C*) Intact expression of MSH2. (*D*) Loss of expression of MSH6. MLH1 and PMS2 are also intact (not shown).

indicate a high likelihood of a germline mutation. Each of the screening tests has advantages and disadvantages. We advocate IHC as a preferred screening method, given the advantages listed previously. If the IHC is abnormal, further testing depends on the pattern of IHC loss. In the event of MLH1/PMS2 loss, *MLH1* promoter methylation analysis is the next step. If methylation is present, the tumor is likely sporadic. In the absence of methylation, *MLH1* mutation analysis should be pursued. *PMS2* mutations are rare; therefore, *PMS2* mutation analysis should be reserved for patients with no detectable *MLH1* mutation. If there is IHC loss of MSH2 and MSH6, mutation analysis for *MSH2* should follow. With isolated MSH6 loss, *MSH6* gene mutation analysis should be pursued.

SOMATIC MUTATIONAL ANALYSIS

Approximately 50% of patients with endometrial cancer with MMR deficiency do not harbor an apparent germline mutation even after epigenetic hypermethylation, germline mutations in *EPCAM*, and inversion of *MSH2* are excluded.[55] The cause

of such discordance can be attributed to unidentified germline mutations, somatic cell mosaicism, a false-positive MMR deficiency test, or biallelic somatic inactivation of the MMR gene(s). Recent evidence based on next-generation sequencing suggests that almost 70% of these patients' tumors harbor 2 acquired somatic (tumor) mutations in MMR genes. Given the screening implications associated with an LS-suspected tumor, somatic mutational analysis and loss of heterozygosity should be considered in the diagnostic evaluation of such patients' tumors. An algorithm that incorporates these testing modalities (Table 2) is provided in Fig. 5.

PROGNOSTIC AND THERAPEUTIC IMPLICATIONS OF MISMATCH REPAIR ABNORMALITIES IN ENDOMETRIAL AND OVARIAN CARCINOMA

The impact of MMR protein status on prognosis and/or therapy in endometrial and ovarian carcinoma is currently unknown. The available data are controversial; some studies have found

Table 2
Testing modalities in Lynch syndrome diagnosis

Assay	Substrate	Position in Workup	Assesses for
MMR IHC	Tumor	Primary screen (preferred)	Loss of ≥1 MMR protein expression (MLH1, PMS2, MSH2, MSH6)
MSI analysis	Tumor	Primary screen (alternative) OR Tertiary test in discordant cases	MSI (a nonspecific by-product of MMR defects)
MLH1 promoter methylation	Tumor	Secondary test	Methylation in MLH1/PMS2-deficient tumors
Germline mutation analysis	Nontumor (typically peripheral blood)	Confirmatory test	Heritable mutations in patients with unmethylated MMR-deficient/MSI-H tumors
Somatic mutation analysis	Tumor	Tertiary test for discordant cases	Somatic mutations in MMR-deficient/MSI-H tumors from patients without detectable germline mutations

Abbreviations: IHC, immunohistochemistry; MMR, mismatch repair; MSI, microsatellite instability; MSI-H, MSI-high.

an association between MMR defects and improved survival, whereas others have shown no association with survival or worse clinical outcomes.[56,57] At least one study has suggested that MMR protein deficiency may warrant alternative therapy for women with ovarian cancer, but this has not been confirmed in independent studies.[58] The Cancer Genome Atlas has identified

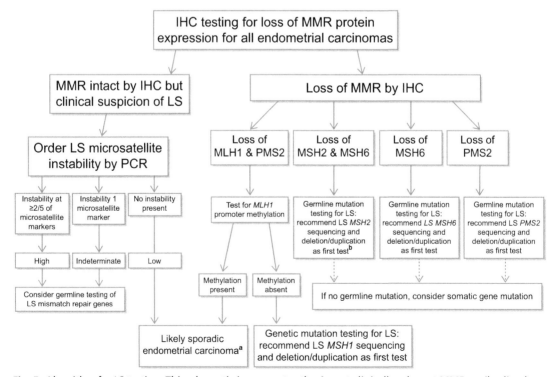

Fig. 5. Algorithm for LS testing. This schematic incorporates the 4 most clinically relevant MMR antibodies, but a 2-antibody approach using PMS2 and MSH6 can also be used as an initial screen. [a] If strong clinical suspicion for LS, consider *MLH1* promoter methylation analysis of non-neoplastic tissue/peripheral blood to evaluate for germline epigenetic *MLH1* promoter methylation. [b] If *MSH2* and *MSH6* unmutated, consider LS *EPCAM*, sequencing, and deletion/duplication.

4 subtypes of endometrial carcinoma on the basis of molecular alterations, 1 of which corresponds to a hypermutated or MSI-H phenotype.[59] Whether molecular subclassification of endometrial carcinomas proves to be more reproducible and clinically relevant than current histomorphologic classifications remains to be determined. Larger controlled studies with long-term clinical follow-up are required to definitively assess the impact of MMR status on therapy and outcome in patients with endometrial and ovarian carcinoma.

SURVEILLANCE AND RISK-REDUCING STRATEGIES FOR ENDOMETRIAL AND OVARIAN CARCINOMAS IN LYNCH SYNDROME

Gynecologic cancer surveillance in LS includes annual pelvic examination with Pap smear, transvaginal ultrasound, pelvic ultrasound, and endometrial biopsy with or without hysteroscopy starting at age 30 to 35 years. The recommended age for commencing surveillance depends on the germline mutation involved and earliest age of onset of cancer in the affected patient's family. However, these surveillance measures have not shown clinical benefits, and cases of interval endometrial carcinomas not detected by surveillance have been reported.[49] The effect of chemoprevention with oral contraceptives in the setting of LS is currently unknown and untested. Risk-reducing hysterectomy and bilateral salpingo-oophorectomy after age 35 years or once childbearing is complete can prevent development of endometrial and ovarian cancer in women with LS due to mutations in *MSH2*, *MSH6*, and *MLH1*.[60] Risk-reducing surgery may not be indicated for LS women with *PMS2* germline mutations due to the currently low observed mortality.[35] However, for those at significant risk for developing a potentially lethal cancer, risk-reducing surgery has been shown to be a more effective and comparatively less expensive option compared with gynecologic surveillance in LS. Because these patients are at risk for occult endometrial and/or ovarian cancer, they should be consented for staging should there be intraoperative evidence of carcinoma. Disadvantages of risk-reducing surgery include surgical complications and induction of surgical menopause. There are no standardized guidelines for evaluating the risk-reducing hysterectomy and/or oophorectomy performed for LS; many of the larger tertiary care cancer institutions submit the entire endometrium, including lower uterine segment and adnexa for microscopic examination.

SUMMARY

LS confers a significant increased lifetime risk for endometrial cancer and ovarian cancer in addition to an increased risk for colorectal and other cancers in affected women. Recent data using universal screening of endometrial cancers indicates that germline mutations may occur in up to 5.9% of unselected women, which is higher than expected based on historic screening algorithms based on personal or family history and/or tumor characteristics. Screening strategies for patients with endometrial cancer have not been as well established as those for colorectal cancer, but IHC is emerging as the preferred screening test for female genital tract tumors based on cost, ease of interpretation, and ability to direct sequencing analysis should an abnormality be detected. Preliminary experience with IHC universal screening of endometrial cancers suggests there may be a higher acceptance of genetic counseling with resultant higher rates of genetic testing compared with referral based on risk factors alone.[61] Nevertheless, a significant proportion of tumors with abnormal IHC tests will ultimately prove to harbor epigenetic hypermethylation or biallelic somatic mutation (or loss of heterozygosity); future LS algorithms should incorporate routine somatic mutation testing as well as methylation testing to guide genetic counseling for these patients and their at-risk relatives.

REFERENCES

1. Aarnio M, Sankila R, Pukkala E, et al. Cancer risk in mutation carriers of DNA-mismatch-repair genes. Int J Cancer 1999;81:214–8.
2. Vasen HF, Watson P, Mecklin JP, et al. New clinical criteria for hereditary nonpolyposis colorectal cancer (HNPCC, Lynch syndrome) proposed by the International Collaborative group on HNPCC. Gastroenterology 1999;116:1453–6.
3. Watson P, Lynch HT. Extracolonic cancer in hereditary nonpolyposis colorectal cancer. Cancer 1993; 71:677–85.
4. Lu KH, Broaddus RR. Gynecologic cancers in Lynch syndrome/HNPCC. Fam Cancer 2005;4:249–54.
5. Hampel H, Frankel W, Panescu J, et al. Screening for Lynch syndrome (hereditary nonpolyposis colorectal cancer) among endometrial cancer patients. Cancer Res 2006;66:7810–7.
6. Hampel H, Frankel WL, Martin E, et al. Screening for the Lynch syndrome (hereditary nonpolyposis colorectal cancer). N Engl J Med 2005;352:1851–60.

7. Ollikainen M, Abdel-Rahman WM, Moisio AL, et al. Molecular analysis of familial endometrial carcinoma: a manifestation of hereditary nonpolyposis colorectal cancer or a separate syndrome? J Clin Oncol 2005;23:4609–16.

8. Ferguson SE, Aronson M, Pollett A, et al. Performance characteristics of screening strategies for Lynch syndrome in unselected women with newly diagnosed endometrial cancer who have undergone universal germline mutation testing. Cancer 2014; 120:3932–9.

9. Malander S, Rambech E, Kristoffersson U, et al. The contribution of the hereditary nonpolyposis colorectal cancer syndrome to the development of ovarian cancer. Gynecol Oncol 2006;101:238–43.

10. Bewtra C, Watson P, Conway T, et al. Hereditary ovarian cancer: a clinicopathological study. Int J Gynecol Pathol 1992;11:180–7.

11. Bonadona V, Bonaiti B, Olschwang S, et al. Cancer risks associated with germline mutations in MLH1, MSH2, and MSH6 genes in Lynch syndrome. JAMA 2011;305:2304–10.

12. Domanska K, Malander S, Masback A, et al. Ovarian cancer at young age: the contribution of mismatch-repair defects in a population-based series of epithelial ovarian cancer before age 40. Int J Gynecol Cancer 2007;17:789–93.

13. Grindedal EM, Renkonen-Sinisalo L, Vasen H, et al. Survival in women with MMR mutations and ovarian cancer: a multicentre study in Lynch syndrome kindreds. J Med Genet 2010;47:99–102.

14. Jensen KC, Mariappan MR, Putcha GV, et al. Microsatellite instability and mismatch repair protein defects in ovarian epithelial neoplasms in patients 50 years of age and younger. Am J Surg Pathol 2008; 32:1029–37.

15. Ketabi Z, Bartuma K, Bernstein I, et al. Ovarian cancer linked to Lynch syndrome typically presents as early-onset, non-serous epithelial tumors. Gynecol Oncol 2011;121:462–5.

16. Watson P, Butzow R, Lynch HT, et al. The clinical features of ovarian cancer in hereditary nonpolyposis colorectal cancer. Gynecol Oncol 2001;82: 223–8.

17. Buttin BM, Powell MA, Mutch DG, et al. Increased risk for hereditary nonpolyposis colorectal cancer-associated synchronous and metachronous malignancies in patients with microsatellite instability-positive endometrial carcinoma lacking MLH1 promoter methylation. Clin Cancer Res 2004;10:481–90.

18. Peltomaki P, Aaltonen LA, Sistonen P, et al. Genetic mapping of a locus predisposing to human colorectal cancer. Science 1993;260:810–2.

19. Loeb LA. Microsatellite instability: marker of a mutator phenotype in cancer. Cancer Res 1994;54: 5059–63.

20. Esteller M, Levine R, Baylin SB, et al. MLH1 promoter hypermethylation is associated with the microsatellite instability phenotype in sporadic endometrial carcinomas. Oncogene 1998;17:2413–7.

21. Mills AM, Liou S, Ford JM, et al. Lynch syndrome screening should be considered for all patients with newly diagnosed endometrial cancer. Am J Surg Pathol 2014;38:1501–9.

22. Westin SN, Lacour RA, Urbauer DL, et al. Carcinoma of the lower uterine segment: a newly described association with Lynch syndrome. J Clin Oncol 2008; 26:5965–71.

23. Broaddus RR, Lynch HT, Chen LM, et al. Pathologic features of endometrial carcinoma associated with HNPCC: a comparison with sporadic endometrial carcinoma. Cancer 2006;106:87–94.

24. Carcangiu ML, Radice P, Casalini P, et al. Lynch syndrome–related endometrial carcinomas show a high frequency of nonendometrioid types and of high FIGO grade endometrioid types. Int J Surg Pathol 2010;18:21–6.

25. Garg K, Leitao MM Jr, Kauff ND, et al. Selection of endometrial carcinomas for DNA mismatch repair protein immunohistochemistry using patient age and tumor morphology enhances detection of mismatch repair abnormalities. Am J Surg Pathol 2009;33:925–33.

26. Honore LH, Hanson J, Andrew SE. Microsatellite instability in endometrioid endometrial carcinoma: correlation with clinically relevant pathologic variables. Int J Gynecol Cancer 2006;16:1386–92.

27. Ryan P, Mulligan AM, Aronson M, et al. Comparison of clinical schemas and morphologic features in predicting Lynch syndrome in mutation-positive patients with endometrial cancer encountered in the context of familial gastrointestinal cancer registries. Cancer 2012;118:681–8.

28. Shia J, Black D, Hummer AJ, et al. Routinely assessed morphological features correlate with microsatellite instability status in endometrial cancer. Hum Pathol 2008;39:116–25.

29. Kwon JS, Scott JL, Gilks CB, et al. Testing women with endometrial cancer to detect Lynch syndrome. J Clin Oncol 2011;29:2247–52.

30. Altrabulsi B, Malpica A, Deavers MT, et al. Undifferentiated carcinoma of the endometrium. Am J Surg Pathol 2005;29:1316–21.

31. Silva EG, Deavers MT, Bodurka DC, et al. Association of low-grade endometrioid carcinoma of the uterus and ovary with undifferentiated carcinoma: a new type of dedifferentiated carcinoma? Int J Gynecol Pathol 2006;25:52–8.

32. Tafe LJ, Garg K, Chew I, et al. Endometrial and ovarian carcinomas with undifferentiated components: clinically aggressive and frequently underrecognized neoplasms. Mod Pathol 2010;23: 781–9.

33. Garg K, Soslow RA. Lynch syndrome (hereditary non-polyposis colorectal cancer) and endometrial carcinoma. J Clin Pathol 2009;62:679–84.

34. Mills AM, Liou S, Kong CS, et al. Are women with endocervical adenocarcinoma at risk for Lynch syndrome? Evaluation of 101 cases including unusual subtypes and lower uterine segment tumors. Int J Gynecol Pathol 2012;31:463–9.

35. ten Broeke SW, Brohet RM, Tops CM, et al. Lynch syndrome caused by germline PMS2 mutations: delineating the cancer risk. J Clin Oncol 2015;33: 319–25.

36. Umar A, Boland CR, Terdiman JP, et al. Revised Bethesda Guidelines for hereditary nonpolyposis colorectal cancer (Lynch syndrome) and microsatellite instability. J Natl Cancer Inst 2004;96:261–8.

37. Vasen HF, Mecklin JP, Khan PM, et al. The International Collaborative Group on Hereditary Non-Polyposis Colorectal Cancer (ICG-HNPCC). Dis Colon Rectum 1991;34:424–5.

38. Lancaster JM, Powell CB, Chen LM, et al. Society of Gynecologic Oncology statement on risk assessment for inherited gynecologic cancer predispositions. Gynecol Oncol 2015;136:3–7.

39. Leenen CH, van Lier MG, van Doorn HC, et al. Prospective evaluation of molecular screening for Lynch syndrome in patients with endometrial cancer </= 70 years. Gynecol Oncol 2012;125:414–20.

40. Mvundura M, Grosse SD, Hampel H, et al. The cost-effectiveness of genetic testing strategies for Lynch syndrome among newly diagnosed patients with colorectal cancer. Genet Med 2010;12:93–104.

41. Evaluation of Genomic Applications in Practice and Prevention (EGAPP) Working Group. Recommendations from the EGAPP Working Group: genetic testing strategies in newly diagnosed individuals with colorectal cancer aimed at reducing morbidity and mortality from Lynch syndrome in relatives. Genet Med 2009;11:35–41.

42. Mojtahed A, Schrijver I, Ford JM, et al. A two-antibody mismatch repair protein immunohistochemistry screening approach for colorectal carcinomas, skin sebaceous tumors, and gynecologic tract carcinomas. Mod Pathol 2011;24: 1004–14.

43. Shia J, Tang LH, Vakiani E, et al. Immunohistochemistry as first-line screening for detecting colorectal cancer patients at risk for hereditary nonpolyposis colorectal cancer syndrome: a 2-antibody panel may be as predictive as a 4-antibody panel. Am J Surg Pathol 2009;33:1639–45.

44. Modica I, Soslow RA, Black D, et al. Utility of immunohistochemistry in predicting microsatellite instability in endometrial carcinoma. Am J Surg Pathol 2007;31:744–51.

45. Geurts-Giele WR, Leenen CH, Dubbink HJ, et al. Somatic aberrations of mismatch repair genes as a cause of microsatellite-unstable cancers. J Pathol 2014;234:548–59.

46. Haraldsdottir S, Hampel H, Tomsic J, et al. Colon and endometrial cancers with mismatch repair deficiency can arise from somatic, rather than germline, mutations. Gastroenterology 2014;147:1308–16.e1.

47. Mills A, Sloan E, Thomas M, et al. Clinicopathologic comparison of Lynch syndrome-associated and Lynch-like endometrial carcinomas identified on universal screening. Am J Surg Pathol 2015;40(2): 155–65.

48. Hagen CE, Lefferts J, Hornick JL, et al. "Null pattern" of immunoreactivity in a Lynch syndrome-associated colon cancer due to germline MSH2 mutation and somatic MLH1 hypermethylation. Am J Surg Pathol 2011;35:1902–5.

49. Resnick K, Straughn JM Jr, Backes F, et al. Lynch syndrome screening strategies among newly diagnosed endometrial cancer patients. Obstet Gynecol 2009;114:530–6.

50. Boland CR, Thibodeau SN, Hamilton SR, et al. A National Cancer Institute Workshop on Microsatellite Instability for cancer detection and familial predisposition: development of international criteria for the determination of microsatellite instability in colorectal cancer. Cancer Res 1998;58:5248–57.

51. Suraweera N, Duval A, Reperant M, et al. Evaluation of tumor microsatellite instability using five quasimonomorphic mononucleotide repeats and pentaplex PCR. Gastroenterology 2002;123:1804–11.

52. McConechy MK, Talhouk A, Li-Chang HH, et al. Detection of DNA mismatch repair (MMR) deficiencies by immunohistochemistry can effectively diagnose the microsatellite instability (MSI) phenotype in endometrial carcinomas. Gynecol Oncol 2015;137:306–10.

53. Bessa X, Balleste B, Andreu M, et al. A prospective, multicenter, population-based study of BRAF mutational analysis for Lynch syndrome screening. Clin Gastroenterol Hepatol 2008;6:206–14.

54. Kawaguchi M, Yanokura M, Banno K, et al. Analysis of a correlation between the BRAF V600E mutation and abnormal DNA mismatch repair in patients with sporadic endometrial cancer. Int J Oncol 2009;34:1541–7.

55. Buchanan DD, Rosty C, Clendenning M, et al. Clinical problems of colorectal cancer and endometrial cancer cases with unknown cause of tumor mismatch repair deficiency (suspected Lynch syndrome). Appl Clin Genet 2014;7:183–93.

56. Fiumicino S, Ercoli A, Ferrandina G, et al. Microsatellite instability is an independent indicator of recurrence in sporadic stage I-II endometrial adenocarcinoma. J Clin Oncol 2001;19:1008–14.

57. Zighelboim I, Goodfellow PJ, Gao F, et al. Microsatellite instability and epigenetic inactivation of MLH1 and outcome of patients with endometrial

carcinomas of the endometrioid type. J Clin Oncol 2007;25:2042–8.

58. Xiao X, Melton DW, Gourley C. Mismatch repair deficiency in ovarian cancer–molecular characteristics and clinical implications. Gynecol Oncol 2014;132: 506–12.

59. Kandoth C, Schultz N, Cherniack AD, et al. Integrated genomic characterization of endometrial carcinoma. Nature 2013;497:67–73.

60. Schmeler KM, Lynch HT, Chen LM, et al. Prophylactic surgery to reduce the risk of gynecologic cancers in the Lynch syndrome. N Engl J Med 2006;354: 261–9.

61. Frolova AI, Babb SA, Zantow E, et al. Impact of an immunohistochemistry-based universal screening protocol for Lynch syndrome in endometrial cancer on genetic counseling and testing. Gynecol Oncol 2015;137:7–13.

Small-Cell Carcinoma of the Ovary of Hypercalcemic Type (Malignant Rhabdoid Tumor of the Ovary)

A Review with Recent Developments on Pathogenesis

Leora Witkowski, BSc[a], Catherine Goudie, MD[b],
William D. Foulkes, MBBS, PhD[a],
W. Glenn McCluggage, FRCPath[c],*

KEYWORDS

- Ovary • Small cell carcinoma of hypercalcemic type • *SMARCA4* • Immunohistochemistry
- Molecular genetics • Mutation

Key points

- Small-cell carcinoma of the ovary of hypercalcemic type (SCCOHT) is a highly malignant and aggressive tumor and represents the most common undifferentiated ovarian malignancy to occur in women younger than 40 years.

- SCCOHT is characterized by deleterious germline or somatic mutations in a single gene, *SMARCA4*, in almost all cases.

- Given the striking morphologic and molecular similarities between SCCOHT and atypical teratoid/malignant rhabdoid tumor, it is clear that SCCOHT is a malignancy of mesenchymal differentiation and a form of ovarian malignant rhabdoid tumor.

- SMARCA4 (BRG1) immunohistochemistry is useful in the diagnosis of SCCOHT because there is loss of nuclear immunoreactivity in this neoplasm but retention of staining in mimics.

ABSTRACT

Small-cell carcinoma of the ovary of hypercalcemic type (SCCOHT) is a highly malignant and aggressive tumor and is the most common undifferentiated ovarian malignancy to occur in women younger than 40. SCCOHT is characterized by deleterious germline or somatic mutations in *SMARCA4*. Given the striking morphologic and molecular similarities between SCCOHT and atypical teratoid/malignant rhabdoid tumor, we propose this should be reflected in a nomenclature change and that SCCOHT be renamed malignant rhabdoid tumor of the ovary. SMARCA4 (BRG1) immunohistochemistry is useful in diagnosis because there is loss of nuclear immunoreactivity in SCCOHT but retention of staining in mimics.

Disclosures: There are no commercial or financial conflicts of interest.
[a] Department of Human Genetics, McGill University, 3755 Cote Ste Catherine, Montreal, Quebec H3T1E2, Canada; [b] Department of Pediatric Oncology, McGill University, 3755 Cote Ste Catherine, Montreal, Quebec H3T1E2, Canada; [c] Department of Pathology, Royal Group of Hospitals Trust, Belfast Health and Social Care Trust, Grosvenor Road, Belfast, Northern Ireland BT12 6BA, UK
* Corresponding author.
E-mail address: glenn.mccluggage@belfasttrust.hscni.net

Surgical Pathology 9 (2016) 215–226
http://dx.doi.org/10.1016/j.path.2016.01.005
1875-9181/16/$ – see front matter © 2016 Elsevier Inc. All rights reserved

OVERVIEW AND HISTORY OF THE DISEASE

Small-cell carcinoma of the ovary of hypercalcemic type (SCCOHT) is a highly malignant undifferentiated ovarian malignancy that was initially described in 1979 by Robert E. Scully.[1] It was characterized by (1) the dominant appearance of small, hyperchromatic cells with brisk mitotic activity, (2) an early age of onset, and (3) the presence of hypercalcemia.[2] Initially, this was considered to most likely represent an epithelial malignancy (carcinoma), although an epithelial histogenesis was never proven, and the term SCCOHT was used to distinguish this type of small-cell "carcinoma" from the neuroendocrine or pulmonary type, which it can resemble.[2,3] The differential diagnosis of SCCOHT may be wide (discussed later) and, along with microscopy, immunohistochemical studies may be necessary to distinguish it from other ovarian neoplasms, although up until recently there has been no specific marker of SCCOHT.

In a seminal study of 150 cases, the mean age at diagnosis was 23.9 years, and 62% of the patients had preoperative hypercalcaemia.[4] Half of the tumors contained a component of large cells with abundant eosinophilic cytoplasm, the so-called "large-cell variant of SCCOHT." Among several interesting features, each of the 23 cases studied by flow cytometry in this study were diploid, an unusual feature for a highly malignant neoplasm.[4] Until recently, the histogenesis of SCCOHT has remained elusive; epithelial, sex cord, germ cell, and neuroendocrine differentiation has been speculated but none proven. Moreover, the underlying molecular events in SCCOHT also were not known until recently, despite the description of a further 250 cases in the English literature and a detailed immunohistochemical study of a series of 15 cases.[5]

In this review, we discuss the clinical and pathologic aspects of SCCOHT, including the differential diagnosis. We also review exciting new data regarding the molecular events underlying this enigmatic neoplasm and present evidence that SCCOHT is a mesenchymal malignancy and a form of ovarian malignant rhabdoid tumor. We propose that this should be reflected in a nomenclature change and that SCCOHT be renamed malignant rhabdoid tumor of the ovary (Box 1).

CLINICAL PRESENTATION AND OUTCOME

Although rare, SCCOHT is the most common undifferentiated ovarian malignancy to occur in women younger than 40.[4] Patients are generally diagnosed in their second or third decade of life (peak between 18 and 30 years), although SCCOHT has been seen in a girl as young as 14 months and a woman as old as 47 years.[4,6–8] Occasional familial cases have been reported.[9,10] The symptoms are usually nonspecific and those related to an abdominal or pelvic mass, but in one-third of cases the patient presents with signs or symptoms of hypercalcemia; as already discussed, approximately two-thirds of patients have increased serum calcium. More than half of patients have extraovarian disease at presentation; this usually comprises local spread to the abdomen and pelvis, but occasionally there is hematogenous spread to distant sites.

SCCOHT has a very poor prognosis, with a 33% survival rate when diagnosed at an early stage and a much more dismal prognosis with advanced

---

Box 1
Key features of small-cell carcinoma of the ovary of hypercalcemic type (SCCOHT)

Clinical

- Patient is typically younger than 50

- Patient may or may not have serum hypercalcemia

Genetic

- 1 Germline *SMARCA4* mutation + 1 somatic mutation or Loss of Heterozygosity (LOH) in the tumor, affecting the other allele

- 1 Somatic *SMARCA4* mutation + LOH in the tumor, affecting the other allele

- Biallelic somatic *SMARCA4* mutations

Histologic

- Typically small cells with scant cytoplasm but there may be a minor, predominant or exclusive component of large cells with abundant eosinophilic cytoplasm and a rhabdoid appearance

- Loss of SMARCA4/BRG1 nuclear staining by immunohistochemistry

stage at diagnosis.[4,6–8] Increased age at diagnosis, normal serum calcium at presentation, no large cell component, small tumors (<10 cm), and the administration of adjuvant radiotherapy have all been found to be favorable prognostic parameters.[4,6–8]

PATHOLOGY OF SMALL-CELL CARCINOMA OF THE OVARY OF HYPERCALCEMIC TYPE

In a large majority of cases, the tumor is unilateral, although familial cases may be bilateral. Macroscopically, these are usually large predominantly solid white or cream-colored neoplasms, often with cystic foci; rare neoplasms are predominantly cystic (Fig. 1). Areas of hemorrhage and necrosis are common.

Histologic examination generally reveals a relatively monotonous appearance with tumor cells arranged in various architectural patterns.[4] The most common, and the one that usually predominates, is a diffuse sheeted pattern, but the neoplastic cells also occasionally grow in nests, cords, or trabeculae (Fig. 2). Follicle-like structures containing eosinophilic, or rarely basophilic, fluid are present in 80% of cases (Fig. 3) and are a characteristic, but not pathognomonic, histologic feature.[4] The tumor cells usually contain round to ovoid hyperchromatic nuclei with minimal cytoplasm resulting in a "small round blue cell" appearance. There are easily identifiable mitotic figures and necrosis is common. In up to 50% of cases,

a component of large cells with abundant eosinophilic cytoplasm is present either as a focal, predominant, or exclusive finding (Fig. 4). When the large cells predominate or are exclusive, this is referred to as the large cell variant of SCCOHT. Typically, the large cells contain abundant glassy eosinophilic cytoplasm and eccentric large pale nuclei with prominent nucleoli, resulting in a rhabdoid appearance.[4] Uncommon morphologic variations, which are usually a focal finding, include a spindle cell component, multinucleate cells, and cells with clear cytoplasm. Mucinous elements, sometimes lining glands or cystic spaces, may also occur and these can be morphologically benign or malignant and even include signet-ring cells. Usually the tumor stroma is minimal and inconspicuous, but rarely there is an appreciable amount of fibrous, myxoid, or edematous stroma. Vascular invasion is commonly seen, especially around the periphery of the neoplasm.

There has been a single case report in which an extraovarian neoplasm with the morphologic features and immunohistochemical profile of SCCOHT developed 5 years after removal of an ovarian mucinous borderline tumor of intestinal type.[11]

GENETICS AND HISTOGENESIS OF SMALL-CELL CARCINOMA OF THE OVARY OF HYPERCALCEMIC TYPE

The past few years have witnessed important and exciting developments regarding the genetics and

Fig. 1. Gross specimen of SCCOHT showing cream-colored neoplasm with areas of hemorrhage.

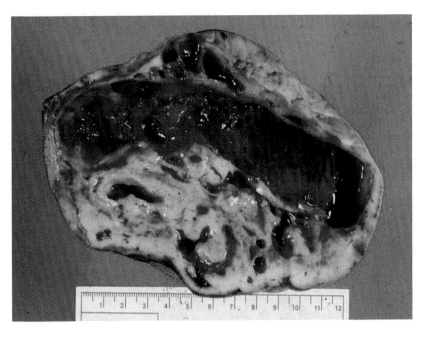

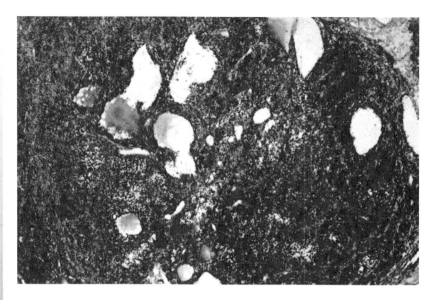

Fig. 2. SCCOHT composed of diffuse sheeted arrangement of small cells with scant cytoplasm, resulting in a small blue cell appearance. Folliclelike structures are present.

molecular events in SCCOHT, which have finally elucidated the histogenesis of this neoplasm. As discussed, in the past epithelial, sex cord, germ cell, and neuroendocrine differentiation has been speculated, but none of these have been proven.[4,5,12] The 2014 World Health Organization (WHO) Classification (as with the previous 2003 Classification) includes SCCOHT within the category of miscellaneous ovarian neoplasms.[13]

Several reports of familial cases of SCCOHT with an autosomal dominant pattern of inheritance have been published, and this provided the initial clue that this could represent a hereditary disorder.[9,10] The rarity of this neoplasm, as well as the lack of available technologies, prevented the discovery of the gene that was causing this potentially hereditary disease until 2014, when 3 separate groups discovered that SCCOHT is a largely monogenic disorder, characterized by deleterious mutations in a single gene, SMARCA4, which encodes the BRG1 protein.[4,14,15] SMARCA4 acts as a tumor suppressor in these neoplasms and

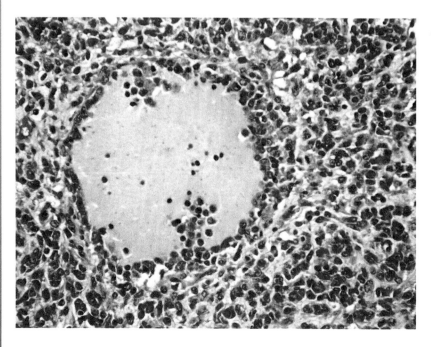

Fig. 3. Folliclelike structures containing eosinophilic or in this case basophilic fluid are a characteristic feature of SCCOHT.

Fig. 4. Large-cell variant of SCCOHT containing cells with large eccentric nuclei and abundant eosinophilic cytoplasm imparting a rhabdoid appearance.

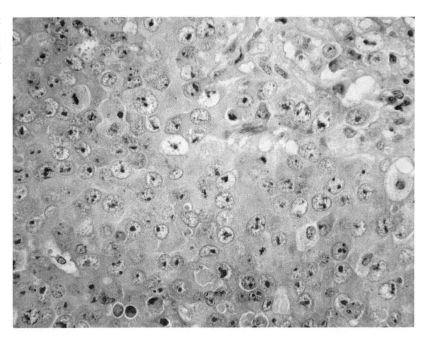

there needs to be loss of both alleles of the gene to develop SCCOHT. This can be in the form of 1 germline and 1 somatic mutation, 2 somatic mutations, or loss of heterozygosity of the wild-type allele in addition to a germline or somatic point mutation, small insertion, or deletion. The mutations in these tumors are most often nonsense or frameshift in type, but occasionally a missense mutation is identified.[4,14,15] Up to half of patients tested have been found to carry a germline mutation, even with no family history of the disease.[6] Due to the rarity of the disease, the penetrance of these germline mutations in the development of SCCOHT is unknown. Currently only one adult woman has been reported to carry a germline mutation in *SMARCA4* without developing the disease; however, she underwent a prophylactic oophorectomy, as 2 of her sisters died of SCCOHT.[16]

The *SMARCA4* gene is part of the SWI/SNF chromatin remodeling complex, which uses ATP to modify chromatin, and includes approximately 20 other genes, many of which have been found to be mutated in cancer. Before the discovery that *SMARCA4* causes SCCOHT, the gene was known to cause rhabdoid tumor predisposition syndrome type 2 (RTPS2) in which, as the name suggests, patients are predisposed to the development of malignant rhabdoid tumors (MRTs).[17] MRTs are pediatric neoplasms that can manifest as either atypical teratoid/rhabdoid tumor (ATRT) in the brain or extracranial MRT; the latter most often develop in the kidney, but can arise in other tissues and organs.[17] In 98% of cases, these neoplasms are caused by

inactivating mutations in *SMARCB1* (also known as *SNF5/INI1/BAF47*), another component of the SWI/SNF complex.[18] The other 2% are caused by mutations in *SMARCA4* (also known as *BRG1*) and, when this is the case, the patients have been reported to have a worse prognosis.[19]

SCCOHT has many morphologic similarities to MRT/ATRT. These include the presence of small cells with scant cytoplasm and, in some cases, the presence of cells with abundant eosinophilic cytoplasm, resulting in a rhabdoid appearance. Due to the genetic and histologic similarity between SCCOHT and MRT/ATRT, our group has suggested that SCCOHT should be renamed MRT of the ovary (MRTO); until such time as this nomenclature is established, the term SCCOHT could be added in parenthesis.[20]

USING IMMUNOHISTOCHEMISTRY TO DIAGNOSE SMALL-CELL CARCINOMA OF THE OVARY OF HYPERCALCEMIC TYPE

A number of older studies investigated the immunophenotype of SCCOHT to try to elucidate the histogenesis, but these studies were inconclusive. The neoplastic cells are sometimes positive with epithelial membrane antigen (EMA), broad-spectrum cytokeratins, WT1, calretinin, and CD10.[5,21–24] Positivity with EMA, cytokeratins, calretinin, and CD10 is generally focal in nature. Most cases exhibit diffuse nuclear positivity with an antibody against the N-terminal of WT1 (**Fig. 5**)[5]; this has

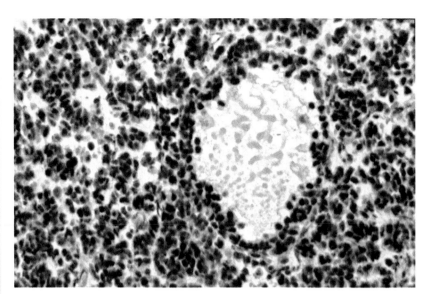

Fig. 5. SCCOHT showing diffuse nuclear staining with WT1.

some diagnostic use, although this marker is positive in many other tumors, including some in the differential diagnosis of SCCOHT. Occasional neoplasms are focally positive with neuroendocrine markers,[5,21–24] and most exhibit diffuse nuclear positivity with p53.[5,23] Desmin, S100, and inhibin are consistently negative. Parathyroid hormone–related protein (PTHRP) has been demonstrated immunohistochemically in some cases of SCCOHT and it has been postulated that this is the explanation for the hypercalcemia in these cases.[24] However, many cases are negative with PTHRP and other neoplasms may be positive, including those not associated with paraneoplastic hypercalcemia.

Given the discovery that *SMARCA4* is mutated in almost all cases of SCCOHT, this has resulted in the development of an antibody that is useful in the diagnosis of this tumor type and distinction from its many mimics. A SMARCA4 (commonly referred to as BRG1) antibody has recently been developed, and in one of the original publications that showed that SCCOHT is characterized by germline and somatic *SMARCA4* mutations, loss of nuclear immunoreactivity with SMARCA4/BRG1 was demonstrated in 51 (94%) of 54 cases.[6] Although there can be technical issues with this antibody resulting in difficulties in interpretation of staining, further studies have shown the value of SMARCA4/BRG1 staining in the diagnosis of SCCOHT.[6,25,26] More than 95% of SCCOHTs exhibit loss of nuclear immunoreactivity with this marker (Fig. 6), making it a potentially important diagnostic tool, although as can be seen, not all cases are negative; one tumor has been reported with loss of SMARCB1 instead SMARCA4.[27] There

also can be heterogeneity of staining in some other neoplasms in the differential diagnosis, but there is usually at least focal retention of nuclear staining.

MANAGEMENT OF SMALL-CELL CARCINOMA OF THE OVARY OF HYPERCALCEMIC TYPE

The traditional management of SCCOHT comprises surgical removal followed by adjuvant chemotherapy. Initial surgical resection remains the baseline for local therapy.[28] In terms of chemotherapy treatment, although the latest report from the European Society for Medical Oncology discussing SCCOHT treatment states that the chemotherapy regimen used is usually akin to that used for small-cell lung cancer, there is no current standard therapy for this rare aggressive ovarian tumor.[29] Multiple adjuvant chemotherapy combinations, mostly including a platinum agent, have been tried, but the prognosis remains dismal. As discussed earlier, stage at diagnosis is the most important factor in determining prognosis.[4,30] Radiation therapy is increasingly being incorporated in a multimodal therapeutic approach for SCCOHT, but its benefit on survival remains inconclusive. Various groups have also included high-dose chemotherapy with stem cell rescue, which has shown encouraging results, even for high-risk patients.[29–31]

CURRENT AND FUTURE RESEARCH

With respect to SCCOHT, no clinical trials have been conducted, presumably due to the rarity of this neoplasm. Several groups recently showed that SMARCA2, the ATPase counterpart of SMARCA4,

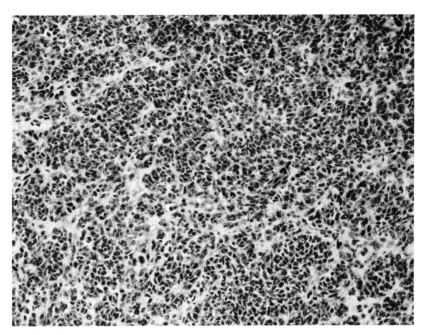

Fig. 6. SCCOHT exhibiting loss of nuclear immunoreactivity with SMARCA4/BRG1; note positive nuclear staining of endothelial cells serving as an internal positive control.

is overexpressed in SMARCA4-deficient tumors and may be a therapeutic target.[32,33] However, in the BIN-67 and SCCOHT-1 cell line, as well as in primary tumours, SMARCA2 is expressed only at the mRNA and not at the protein level.[6] Studies have been conducted in which other drugs and oncolytic viruses were tested in in vitro and in vivo models of SCCOHT,[34,35] but thus far none have reached clinical trials. Due to the genetic similarity between SMARCA4-deficient SCCOHT and SMARCB1-deficient MRTs, it is anticipated that genes dysregulated in SCCOHT will be similar to those in MRTs. As such, future research should focus on determining overexpressed genes in SCCOHT that may be amenable for targeted therapies; this strategy offers some hope in improving the dismal prognosis of SCCOHT.

DIAGNOSTIC/GENETIC TESTING ALGORITHM FOR SMALL-CELL CARCINOMA OF THE OVARY OF HYPERCALCEMIC TYPE

Because SCCOHT is a rare neoplasm such that many or even most individual pathologists will not encounter even a single example in their diagnostic practice in their lifetime, we recommend that a specialist opinion is sought from an expert gynecological pathologist. Because of the difficulty in diagnosing SCCOHT, demonstration of the loss of SMARCA4/BRG1 by immunohistochemistry may be very valuable but is not always necessary.[6,25,26] Given the incidence of germline mutations (up to one-half) that lead to the

development of the tumor, an algorithm for diagnosing SCCOHT and the steps that should be undertaken in terms of genetic testing have been described by our group.[16] (**Box 2**) Briefly, once the diagnosis has been confirmed by a specialist pathologist, which may or may not necessitate SMARCA4/BRG1 immunostaining, the patient should be counseled and germline *SMARCA4* mutation testing undertaken. If the patient does harbor a germline mutation and the neoplasm appears to be unilateral and has been diagnosed following removal of just 1 ovary (as is commonly undertaken in young women), removal of the unaffected ovary should be considered. Additionally, any female family members should be tested for the causative mutation. In the case of no germline mutation, the unaffected ovary can be retained. Somatic genetic testing can be performed on the tumor as necessary to confirm the diagnosis and the absence of a germline mutation. Note that in many cases, loss of the entire short arm of chromosome 19 is seen in the tumor. Due to the semiquantitative nature of Sanger sequencing, this loss may be detectable only by using next-generation sequencing methods.

DIFFERENTIAL DIAGNOSIS OF SMALL-CELL CARCINOMA OF THE OVARY OF HYPERCALCEMIC TYPE

SCCOHT is the prototypical ovarian neoplasm composed predominantly or exclusively of small round cells with scant cytoplasm (so-called "small

---

Box 2
Diagnostic/genetic testing algorithm for SCCOHT

1. Have the tumor reviewed by a gynecological pathologist and the diagnosis confirmed (this may necessitate SMARCA4/BRG1 immunohistochemical staining)

2. Once the diagnosis is confirmed, counsel the patient for germline SMARCA4 sequencing

3. In the case of a germline mutation, consider removal of the unaffected ovary in unilateral SCCOHT if only one ovary has been removed

4. In the case of a germline mutation, test family members for mutation

5. In the case of no germline mutation, if appropriate according to age and clinical context, retain unaffected ovary in unilateral SCCOHT

6. Perform somatic testing on the tumor as necessary

---

round blue cell tumor"). The differential diagnosis of the various neoplasms in this broad group may be wide, and pathologists commonly struggle with these tumors due to overlapping morphology and immunohistochemistry.[36] Many of these tumors occur most commonly in young women, are highly aggressive, and require specific chemotherapeutic agents, which make a correct diagnosis imperative. In diagnosing the various tumor types, immunohistochemistry may be of value as can molecular studies; these are discussed when covering the individual tumor types in the differential diagnosis. Although typical SCCOHT is part of the differential diagnosis of a small round blue cell tumor, the large cell variant of SCCOHT may be confused with a variety of neoplasms composed of large cells, such as undifferentiated carcinoma and malignant melanoma. A selection of neoplasms that enter into the differential diagnosis of SCCOHT are discussed briefly in the next sections.

SEX CORD–STROMAL TUMORS

Both adult granulosa cell tumor (AGCT) and juvenile granulosa cell tumor (JGCT) may enter into the differential diagnosis of SCCOHT. AGCT may be confused with typical SCCOHT, and JGCT may be confused with the large-cell variant. In typical SCCOHT, the nuclei are much more hyperchromatic with greater mitotic activity than in AGCT, which is characterized by angular vesicular nuclei, sometimes with grooves. The follicles are more likely to be intermediate in size in SCCOHT compared with the microfollicular and macrofollicular arrangements characteristic of AGCT. Both the large-cell variant of SCCOHT and JGCT are characterized by the presence of large cells with abundant cytoplasm and by the formation of intermediate-sized folliclelike spaces, often containing eosinophilic or sometimes basophilic

fluid, and there may be a close morphologic resemblance between the two neoplasms. Both neoplasms are typically mitotically active and the nuclei may be hyperchromatic. Pointers in favor of a JGCT include the presence of estrogenic manifestations and normal preoperative serum calcium. Paradoxically, JGCT often exhibits greater nuclear pleomorphism than SCCOHT, sometimes with bizarre nuclear forms, and a theca cell component is often present. In the large-cell variant of SCCOHT, the cells typically have a rhabdoid phenotype with eccentric nuclei and glassy eosinophilic cytoplasm, which is not usually a feature of JGCT.

Immunohistochemistry may be of considerable value in the distinction between SCCOHT on the one hand and AGCT and JGCT on the other. SCCOHT is negative with inhibin, whereas AGCT and JGCT are almost always positive.[37,38] EMA positivity favors SCCOHT because ovarian sex cord–stromal neoplasms are usually negative,[39] although in one study focal EMA positivity was seen in 6 of 12 cases of JGCT.[40] As discussed earlier, there is absence of nuclear SMARCA4/BRG1 immunoreactivity in SCCOHT with retention of staining in AGCT and JGCT.

On occasions, a poorly differentiated Sertoli-Leydig cell tumor or an unclassifiable sex cord–stromal tumor may enter into the differential diagnosis of SCCOHT. However, in the former, extensive sampling often reveals a component of more typical Sertoli-Leydig cell tumor and immunohistochemistry will assist, as discussed in the prior paragraph.

OVARIAN SMALL-CELL CARCINOMA OF PULMONARY TYPE (SMALL-CELL NEUROENDOCRINE CARCINOMA)

Small-cell neuroendocrine carcinoma, identical to that occurring more commonly within the lung, may rarely arise in the ovary.[3] This is referred to in the WHO 2014 Classification as ovarian small-cell carcinoma of pulmonary type[13]; however, the term small-cell neuroendocrine carcinoma appears to be a more appropriate designation. Sometimes these neoplasms occur in association with a component of ovarian carcinoma of one of the usual types, most commonly endometrioid; rarely, such neoplasms arise within a teratoma.[41]

Histologic examination shows small to medium-sized cells with scant cytoplasm and hyperchromatic nuclei. Nuclear molding is often present together with abundant necrosis and apoptosis, the histologic features being identical to small-cell carcinoma of the lung.

Distinction from SCCOHT is facilitated by a combination of features. SCCOHT usually occurs in a younger age group and is often associated with paraneoplastic hypercalcemia. The folliclelike spaces commonly seen in SCCOHT are not usually a feature of pulmonary-type small-cell carcinoma, in which nuclear molding is more common. The identification of a component of a more usual ovarian carcinoma is suggestive of pulmonary-type small-cell carcinoma and extensive pathologic sampling may assist in this regard. Immunohistochemistry may be of value, as pulmonary-type small-cell carcinoma is usually positive with SMARCA4/BRG1 and with neuroendocrine markers, such as chromogranin and synaptophysin, although positive staining with neuroendocrine markers may be focal and occasional cases may be negative. Metastatic small-cell neuroendocrine carcinoma from the lung and other organs occasionally involves the ovary. Obviously, clinical history may be paramount in such cases. TTF1 is usually positive in metastatic lung small-cell neuroendocrine carcinoma but also may be positive in small-cell neuroendocrine carcinomas arising in other organs.[42]

DESMOPLASTIC SMALL ROUND CELL TUMOR

Desmoplastic small round cell tumor (DSRCT) is a rare neoplasm that most commonly occurs in young men (4:1 male-to-female ratio) with a mean age of 25 years.[43,44] The abdominal cavity is the most common site. At presentation, there are usually multiple large tumor nodules with widespread peritoneal involvement. In women, the clinical, radiological, and operative impression may be of an ovarian neoplasm with the distribution simulating bilateral ovarian tumors with widespread peritoneal and omental involvement.[45,46]

Histologic examination typically reveals well-circumscribed solid nodules of tumor cells set in an abundant desmoplastic stroma. In some cases, the stroma is focally inconspicuous and rarely there is myxoid change. The tumor is characterized by a somewhat monomorphic appearance with round to ovoid hyperchromatic nuclei with inconspicuous nucleoli and scant cytoplasm. Mitotic figures are easily identified and areas of necrosis are common. Morphologic variations include the presence of rosettelike, tubular or glandular structures; trabecular arrangements; a spindle-cell component; cells with abundant eosinophilic cytoplasm (sometimes resulting in a rhabdoid appearance); cells with clear cytoplasm; signet-ring cells; and foci of marked nuclear pleomorphism.

DSRCT is characterized by positive staining with a variety of epithelial, neural, and mesenchymal markers.[47] Desmin positivity is especially common (39 of 39 cases in one large study[46]), usually with a globular paranuclear pattern. DSRCT exhibits nuclear staining with an antibody against the C-terminal of WT1, in contrast to SCCOHT, which exhibits nuclear positivity with an antibody against the N-terminal.[48]

DSRCT exhibits a unique chromosomal translocation (t[11;22] [p13;q12]), which results in the EWS/WT1 chimeric transcript, the presence of which is essentially diagnostic of this neoplasm.[49]

EWING FAMILY OF TUMORS

Tumors in the Ewing family (also referred to as peripheral primitive neuroectodermal tumor [pPNET]) have rarely been described within the ovary[50,51] and may mimic SCCOHT because of the predominant component of small cells with scant cytoplasm. Histologic examination reveals similar features to the same tumors in other organs and tissues with sheets or nests of small cells with round to ovoid hyperchromatic nuclei and generally scant cytoplasm. Frequent mitoses and areas of necrosis are often present. Rosettes, which can be sparse or abundant, may be present. Tumors in the Ewing family contain EWSR1 and other variant chromosomal translocations.[50,51]

CD99 is usually positive with membranous immunoreactivity. However, CD99 is not specific for tumors in the Ewing family, and other neoplasms in the broad category of small round cell tumor can be positive, including rhabdomyosarcoma and lymphoma. In one study, all SCCOHTs were CD99 negative.[5] CD99 may be positive in ovarian sex cord–stromal tumors, including AGCT and JGCT.[52] Tumors in the Ewing family are commonly positive with FLI-1 with nuclear immunoreactivity, which may be of value in diagnosis.[53,54] However, FLI-1 also may be positive in other neoplasms, including ovarian sex cord–stromal tumors; for example, one study showed positivity in all cases of JGCT studied.[55]

Somewhat similar neoplasms rarely occur in the ovary as one variant of primary ovarian neuroectodermal tumor. These are rare neoplasms, similar to their counterparts in the central nervous system, and are of 3 main morphologic subtypes: differentiated (most commonly ependymoma but occasionally astrocytoma or oligodendroglioma), anaplastic (resembling glioblastoma multiforme), and primitive (resembling medulloepithelioma, ependymoblastoma, neuroblastoma, or medulloblastoma).[56] Some of these neoplasms arise from teratomas and others may represent monodermal teratomas; the primitive neoplasms are more akin to central PNETs rather than tumors in the Ewing family.[56] In contrast to tumors in the Ewing family, central PNETs are usually CD99 negative.

MISCELLANEOUS NEOPLASMS

A variety of other neoplasms that may arise within or involve the ovary can occasionally mimic SCCOHT.[36] These include low-grade endometrial stromal sarcoma, either primary in the ovary or metastatic from the uterus, and some germ-cell tumors, such as dysgerminoma and immature teratoma. Other small round blue cell tumors, such as malignant lymphoma, rhabdomyosarcoma, and neuroblastoma, may involve the ovary usually secondarily; the morphologic and immunohistochemical features being identical to when these neoplasms involve more common sites. Poorly differentiated or undifferentiated ovarian carcinomas may also enter into the differential diagnosis, especially of the large-cell variant of SCCOHT. Finally, malignant melanoma (primary in the ovary or more commonly metastatic) may enter into the differential. Some malignant melanomas involving the ovary are composed of small cells with scant cytoplasm and even form follicle-like spaces closely mimicking SCCOHT.[57,58] The large-cell variant of SCCOHT may also be confused with malignant melanoma. A history of melanoma, a nested or nevoid pattern, melanin pigment, and the presence of prominent eosinophilic nucleoli or intranuclear inclusions may assist in establishing a diagnosis of melanoma. Immunohistochemical staining with melanoma markers, such as S100, Melan-A, and HMB45, may be of value.

REFERENCES

1. Scully RE. Tumors of the ovary and maldeveloped gonads. In: Hartmann WH, Cowan WR, editors. Atlas of tumor pathology, second series, fascicle 16. Washington, DC: Armed Forces Institute of Pathology; 1979.

2. Dickersin GR, Kline IW, Scully RE. Small cell carcinoma of the ovary with hypercalcemia: a report of eleven cases. Cancer 1982;49:188–97.

3. Eichhorn JH, Young RH, Scully RE. Primary ovarian small cell carcinoma of pulmonary type. A clinicopathologic, immunohistologic, and flow cytometric analysis of 11 cases. Am J Surg Pathol 1992;16:926–38.

4. Young RH, Oliva E, Scully RE. Small-cell carcinoma of the ovary, hypercalcemic type–a clinicopathological analysis of 150 cases. Am J Surg Pathol 1994; 18:1102–16.

5. McCluggage WG, Oliva E, Connolly LE, et al. An immunohistochemical analysis of ovarian small cell carcinoma of hypercalcemic type. Int J Gynecol Pathol 2004;23:330–6.

6. Witkowski L, Carrot-Zhang J, Albrecht S, et al. Germline and somatic SMARCA4 mutations characterize small cell carcinoma of the ovary, hypercalcemic type. Nat Genet 2014;46:438–43.

7. Estel R, Hackethal A, Kalder M, et al. Small cell carcinoma of the ovary of the hypercalcaemic type: an analysis of clinical and prognostic aspects of a rare disease on the basis of cases published in the literature. Arch Gynecol Obstet 2011;284:1277–82.

8. Young RH. Ovarian tumors and tumor-like lesions in the first three decades. Semin Diagn Pathol 2014;31: 382–426.

9. Lamovec J, Bracko M, Cerar O. Familial occurrence of small cell carcinoma of the ovary. Arch Pathol Lab Med 1995;119:523–7.

10. Longy M, Toulouse C, Mage P, et al. Familial cluster of ovarian small cell carcinoma. A new mendelian entity? J Med Genet 1998;33:333–5.

11. Mansor S, Nagarajan S, Sumathi VP, et al. Borderline ovarian mucinous neoplasm recurring as small cell carcinoma of hypercalcemic type: evidence for an epithelial histogenesis and relationship with ovarian mucinous tumors for this enigmatic neoplasm. Int J Gynecol Pathol 2011;30:380–5.

12. Ulbright TM, Roth LM, Stehman FB, et al. Poorly differentiated (small cell) carcinoma of the ovary in young women: evidence supporting a germ cell origin. Hum Pathol 1987;18:175–84.

13. Kurman RJ, Carcangiu ML, Herrington CS, et al, editors. WHO classification of tumours of female reproductive organs. Lyon (France): International Agency for Research on Cancer; 2014.

14. Ramos P, Karnezis AN, Craig DW, et al. Small cell carcinoma of the ovary, hypercalcemic type, displays frequent inactivating germline and somatic mutations in SMARCA4. Nat Genet 2014;46:427–9.

15. Jelinic P, Mueller JJ, Olvera N, et al. Recurrent SMARCA4 mutations in small cell carcinoma of the ovary. Nat Genet 2014;46:424–6.

16. Berchuck A, Witkowski L, Hasselblatt M, et al. Prophylactic oophorectomy for hereditary small cell carcinoma of the ovary, hypercalcemic type. Gynecol Oncol Rep 2015;12:20–2.

17. Brennan B, Stiller C, Bourdeaut F. Extracranial rhabdoid tumours: what we have learned so far and future directions. Lancet Oncol 2013;14: 329–36.

18. Witkowski L, Foulkes WD. In brief: picturing the complex world of chromatin remodelling families. J Pathol 2015;237(4):403–6.

19. Hasselblatt M, Nagel I, Oyen F, et al. SMARCA4-mutated atypical teratoid/rhabdoid tumors are associated with inherited germline alterations and poor prognosis. Acta Neuropathol 2014;128:453–6.

20. Foulkes WD, Clarke BA, Hasselblatt M, et al. No small surprise—small cell carcinoma of the ovary, hypercalcaemic type, is a malignant rhabdoid tumour. J Pathol 2014;233:209–14.

21. Riopel MA, Perlman PJ, Seidman JD, et al. Inhibin and epithelial membrane antigen immunohistochemistry assist in the diagnosis of sex cord-stromal tumors and provide clues to the histogenesis of hypercalcemic small cell carcinomas. Int J Gynecol Pathol 1998;17:46–53.

22. Aguirre P, Thor AD, Scully RE. Ovarian small cell carcinoma. Histogenetic considerations based on immunohistochemical and other findings. Am J Clin Pathol 1989;92:140–9.

23. Seidman J. Small cell carcinoma of the ovary of the hypercalcemic type: p53 protein accumulation and clinicopathologic features. Gynecol Oncol 1995;59: 283–7.

24. Matias-Guiu X, Prat J, Young RH, et al. Human parathyroid hormone-related protein in ovarian small cell carcinoma. An immunohistochemical study. Cancer 1994;73:1878–81.

25. Karanian-Philippe M, Velasco V, Longy M, et al. SMARCA4 (BRG1) loss of expression is a useful marker for the diagnosis of ovarian small cell carcinoma of the hypercalcemic type (ovarian rhabdoid tumor): a comprehensive analysis of 116 rare gynecologic tumors, 9 soft tissue tumors, and 9 melanomas. Am J Surg Pathol 2015;39:1197–205.

26. Agaimy A, Thiel F, Hartmann A, et al. SMARCA4-deficient undifferentiated carcinoma of the ovary (small cell carcinoma, hypercalcemic type): clinicopathologic and immunohistochemical study of 3 cases. Ann Diagn Pathol 2015;19(5):283–7.

27. Ramos P, Karnezis AN, Hendricks WPD, et al. Loss of the tumour suppressor SMARCA4 in small cell carcinoma of the ovary, hypercalcemic type (SCCOHT). Rare Dis 2014;2(1):e967148.

28. Reed N, Millan D, Verheijen R, et al. Non-epithelial ovarian cancer: ESMO clinical practice guidelines for diagnosis, treatment and follow-up. Ann Oncol 2010;21:v31–6.

29. Harrison ML, Hoskins P, du Bois A, et al. Small cell of the ovary, hypercalcemic type—analysis of combined experience and recommendation for management. A GCIG study. Gynecol Oncol 2006;100: 233–8.

30. Distelmaier F, Calaminus G, Harms D, et al. Ovarian small cell carcinoma of the hypercalcemic type in children and adolescents. Cancer 2006;107: 2298–306.

31. Pressey JG, Kelly DR, Hawthorne HT. Successful treatment of preadolescents with small cell carcinoma of the ovary hypercalcemic type. J Pediatr Hematol Oncol 2013;35:566–9.

32. Hoffman GR, Rahal R, Buxton F, et al. Functional epigenetics approach identifies BRM/SMARCA2 as a critical synthetic lethal target in BRG1-deficient cancers. Proc Natl Acad Sci U S A 2014;111: 3128–33.

33. Oike T, Ogiwara H, Tominaga Y, et al. A synthetic lethality–based strategy to treat cancers harboring a genetic deficiency in the chromatin remodeling factor BRG1. Cancer Res 2013;73:5508–18.

34. Gamwell L, Gambaro K, Merziotis M, et al. Small cell ovarian carcinoma: genomic stability and responsiveness to therapeutics. Orphanet J Rare Dis 2013;8:33.

35. Otte A, Rauprich F, Hillemanns P, et al. In vitro and in vivo therapeutic approach for a small cell carcinoma of the ovary hypercalcaemic type using a SCCOHT-1 cellular model. Orphanet J Rare Dis 2014;9:126.

36. McCluggage WG. Ovarian neoplasms composed of small round cells: a review. Adv Anat Pathol 2004; 11:288–96.

37. Deavers MT, Malpica A, Liu J, et al. Ovarian sex cord-stromal tumors: an immunohistochemical study including a comparison of calretinin and inhibin. Mod Pathol 2003;16:584–90.

38. McCluggage WG, Maxwell P, Sloan JM. Immunohistochemical staining of ovarian granulosa cell tumors with monoclonal antibody against inhibin. Hum Pathol 1997;28:1034–8.

39. Costa MJ, De Rose PB, Roth LM, et al. Immunohistochemical phenotype of ovarian granulosa cell tumors: absence of epithelial membrane antigen has diagnostic value. Hum Pathol 1994;25:60–6.

40. McCluggage WG. Immunoreactivity of ovarian juvenile granulosa cell tumours with epithelial membrane antigen. Histopathology 2005;46:235–6.

41. Lim SC, Choi JJ, Suh CH. A case of small cell carcinoma arising in mature cystic teratoma of the ovary. Pathol Int 1998;48:834–9.

42. McCluggage WG, Kennedy K, Busam KJ. An immunohistochemical study of cervical neuroendocrine carcinomas: neoplasms that are commonly TTF1 positive and which may express CK20 and P63. Am J Surg Pathol 2010;34:525–32.

43. Ordonez NG. Desmoplastic small round cell tumor. I: a histopathologic study of 39 cases with emphasis on unusual histological patterns. Am J Surg Pathol 1998;22:1303–13.

44. Gerald WL, Miller HK, Battifora H, et al. Intra-abdominal desmoplastic small round cell tumor. Report of 19 cases of a distinctive type of high grade polyphenotypic malignancy affecting young individuals. Am J Surg Pathol 1991;15:499–513.

45. Parker LP, Duong JL, Wharton JT, et al. Desmoplastic small round cell tumor: report of a case presenting as a primary ovarian neoplasm. Eur J Gynaecol Oncol 2002;23:199–202.

46. Young RH, Eichhorn JH, Dickersin GR, et al. Ovarian involvement by the intra-abdominal desmoplastic small round cell tumor with divergent differentiation: a report of three cases. Hum Pathol 1992;23:454–64.

47. Ordonez NG. Desmoplastic small round cell tumor: II: an ultrastructural and immunohistochemical study with emphasis on new immunohistochemical markers. Am J Surg Pathol 1998;22:1314–27.

48. McCluggage WG. WT-1 immunohistochemical expression in small round blue cell tumours. Histopathology 2008;52:631–2.

49. Gerald WL, Rosai J, Ladayni M. Characterisation of the genomic breakpoint and chimeric transcripts in the EWS-WT1 gene fusion of desmoplastic small round cell tumor. Proc Natl Acad Sci U S A 1995;92:1028–32.

50. Kawachi S, Fukuda T, Miyamoto S, et al. Peripheral primitive neuroectodermal tumor of the ovary confirmed by CD99 immunostaining, karyotypic analysis and RT-PCR for EWS/FLI-1 chimeric mRNA. Am J Surg Pathol 1998;22:1417–22.

51. Kim KJ, Jang BW, Lee SK, et al. A case of peripheral primitive neuroectodermal tumor of the ovary. Int J Gynecol Cancer 2004;14:370–2.

52. Loo KT, Leung AKF, Chan JKC. Immunohistochemical staining of ovarian granulosa cell tumours with MIC2 antibody. Histopathology 1995;27:388–90.

53. Folpe AL, Hill CE, Parham DM, et al. Immunohistochemical detection of FLI-1 protein expression: a study of 132 round cell tumors with emphasis on CD99-positive mimics of Ewing's sarcoma/primitive neuroectodermal tumor. Am J Surg Pathol 2000;24:1657–62.

54. Rossi S, Orvieto E, Furlanetto A, et al. Utility of the immunohistochemical detection of FLI-1 expression in round cell and vascular neoplasm using a monoclonal antibody. Mod Pathol 2004;17:547–52.

55. Jarboe EA, Hirschowitz SL, Geiersbach KB, et al. Juvenile granulosa cell tumors: immunoreactivity for CD99 and Fli-1 and EWSR1 translocation status: a study of 11 cases. Int J Gynecol Pathol 2014;33:11–5.

56. Kleinman GM, Young RH, Scully RE. Primary neuroectodermal tumors of the ovary. A report of 25 cases. Am J Surg Pathol 1993;17:764–78.

57. Young RH, Scully RE. Malignant melanoma metastatic to the ovary: a clinicopathologic analysis of 20 cases. Am J Surg Pathol 1991;15:849–60.

58. McCluggage WG, Bissonnette JP, Young RH. Primary malignant melanoma of the ovary: a report of 9 definite or probable cases with emphasis on their morphologic diversity and mimicry of other primary and secondary ovarian neoplasms. Int J Gynecol Pathol 2006;25:321–9.

Gynecologic Manifestations of the DICER1 Syndrome

Colin J.R. Stewart, FRCPA[a],*, Adrian Charles, FRCPA[b],
William D. Foulkes, PhD[c,d,e,f]

KEYWORDS

- DICER1 • Syndrome • Mutation • Sertoli-Leydig cell tumor • Ovary • Cervix • Rhabdomyosarcoma

Key points

- Patients with germline DICER1 mutations are predisposed to a wide range of relatively rare tumors.
- In the female genital tract, ovarian sex cord–stromal tumors and cervical embryonal rhabdomyosarcoma are most common.
- The tumors may show morphologic differences compared with their sporadic counterparts.
- Genetic evaluation should be considered in patients presenting with these tumors.

ABSTRACT

Patients with germline *DICER1* mutations are at increased risk of developing a wide range of tumors, most of which are relatively rare in the general population. In the gynecologic tract, these include ovarian sex cord–stromal tumors, particularly Sertoli-Leydig cell tumor, and embryonal rhabdomyosarcoma of the cervix. In some cases, these are the sentinel neoplasms. DICER1-associated tumors may have distinctive morphologic appearances that may prompt the pathologist to consider an underlying tumor predisposition syndrome and therefore consideration of genetic evaluation in the patient and her family.

MOLECULAR OVERVIEW OF DICER1

The highly conserved RNase III enzyme Dicer (DICER1 in *Homo sapiens*) is critical for the biogenesis of most small RNAs. Following Dicer's discovery, several key studies demonstrated Dicer's importance in both physiologic and pathologic states.[1–5] Structural studies on the full-length protein, fragments, and domains of Dicer have clarified how double-stranded (ds) RNA precursors such as long dsRNA or pre-microRNAs dock on the enzyme and will lead to further critical insights. From a cancer perspective, initial studies focused on expression levels of Dicer and other microRNA processing factors but these are difficult to interpret and are not discussed further here. The

Conflicts of Interest and Funding Sources: The authors have no conflicts of interest. Work in Dr W.D. Foulkes's laboratory on DICER1 has been supported by grants from Alex's Lemonade Stand Foundation and the Canadian Cancer Society Research Institute.
[a] Department of Histopathology, King Edward Memorial Hospital, School for Women's and Infants' Health, University of Western Australia, Subiaco, Perth, Western Australia 6008, Australia; [b] Department of Anatomical Pathology, Sidra Medical and Research Center, PO Box 26999, Doha, Qatar; [c] Department of Human Genetics, McGill University, Montreal, Quebec, Canada; [d] Department of Oncology, McGill University, Montreal, Quebec, Canada; [e] Department of Medical Genetics, Jewish General Hospital, McGill University Health Centre, Montreal, Quebec, Canada; [f] Cancer Genetics Laboratory, Lady Davis Institute, Montreal, Quebec H3T 1E2, Canada
* Corresponding author.
E-mail address: colin.stewart@health.wa.gov.au

work described in this paragraph is summarized in a recent review.[6]

Dicer1 knockout embryos are incompatible with life and usually Dicer1-null embryonic stem (ES) cells could not be generated.[7,8] However, using special conditions, Dicer1-null ES can be generated and although they exhibit normal morphology they fail to differentiate.[9] Given the catastrophic effect of complete loss of Dicer1 on mammalian ES development it is perhaps surprising that humans carrying a DICER1 mutation on one allele are often normal (see next paragraph).

The key clinical features of the DICER1 syndrome (OMIM #601200), were first recognized in 1996.[10] However, it was not until 2009 that deleterious DICER1 mutations were identified in the families with the phenotypes that had led to its earlier recognition as a discrete familial entity.[11] One of the reasons that it took a relatively long time to molecularly identify this syndrome is because, with the exception of multinodular goiter (MNG, which was identified as part of the syndrome later), the benign and malignant tumors that comprise the syndrome are rare to ultrarare, and the syndrome has a very variable penetrance. Most of the conditions present at some point between birth and age 30 years, but more recently later presentations have been noted. The risk of developing any of the listed conditions is quite low and, overall, fewer than half of all mutation carriers are estimated to be clinically affected. Furthermore, although the most typical clinical presentations of DICER1 mutations are listed under "Key Features of the DICER1 Syndrome," the syndrome is notably pleiotropic, including other highly characteristic but exceptionally rare conditions such as pituitary blastoma and anaplastic renal sarcoma, as well as rare ocular and sinonasal tumors.[6] Other generally more common conditions such as Wilms tumor have also been reported in mutation carriers.[6]

Pitfalls
IN THE DIAGNOSIS OF
DICER1 SYNDROME

! Type 1 PPB can be confused with a congenital cystic adenomatoid malformation

! MNG may be evident only on ultrasound examination and therefore can be overlooked

! Cystic nephroma can be misdiagnosed as a simple renal cyst and can occur later in childhood

! Many of the rarer tumors have been previously misinterpreted as other conditions

From a molecular standpoint, the DICER1 syndrome has a number of unusual features. It was the first gene in which germline mutations affecting microRNA maturation (ie, the processing of precursor microRNAs to their mature counterparts) were found to be associated with human tumors.[11] These mutations were found to be typical of a tumor suppressor gene in that in general they partially or completely disable one allele of the DICER1 gene.[11] Usually, tumor suppressor genes require "2 hits" to be rendered sufficiently nonfunctional to permit a tumor to arise.[12] "Second hits" following the initial germline mutation do indeed occur in DICER1-related tumors, but highly unusually they are limited to restricted regions of the DICER1 sequence that code for the RNase IIIb endonuclease function.[13,14] This domain normally functions to cleave precursor microRNAs to their final mature length. Moreover, these mutations are nearly always a single base substitution leading to an amino acid change,[13] which in contrast to the initial hit functionally impairs the protein without overall protein loss.[11]

Key Features
OF THE DICER1 SYNDROME

Personal or family history of unusual childhood/adolescent tumors such as the following:
• Pleuropulmonary blastoma (PPB) arising before age 6 years

• Multinodular goiter (MNG) in a child or adolescent

• Cystic nephroma, usually before 4 years of age

• Ovarian sex cord–stromal tumors

• Embryonal rhabdomyosarcoma (ERMS) of the cervix

• Other rare tumors, including pituitary blastoma, nasal chondromesenchymal hamartoma, ciliary body (and occasionally cerebral) medulloepithelioma, juvenile hamartomatous intestinal polyps, bladder ERMS in early childhood, primitive neuroectodermal tumor/Ewing sarcoma

The female genital tract neoplasms most closely linked with DICER1 syndrome are ovarian sex cord–stromal tumors (SCST) and cervical embryonal rhabdomyosarcoma (cERMS), but other possible gynecologic tumor associations are discussed briefly.

OVARIAN SEX CORD–STROMAL TUMORS

BACKGROUND AND CLINICAL FEATURES

Key features of ovarian SCST in the DICER1 syndrome are summarized in the "Key Features" box. Inclusion of ovarian SCST in the DICER1 syndrome was established by 3 studies published in 2011.[15–17] An analysis of 325 individuals from the International Pleuropulmonary Blastoma (PPB) Registry identified ovarian SCST in 12 patients who had a personal or family history of PPB or of PPB-related neoplasms.[15] The mean age was 12.3 years (range 2–32 years). Rio Frio and colleagues[16] reported 3 individuals, aged 14, 18, and 32 years, with germline DICER1 mutations, familial MNG, and ovarian Sertoli-Leydig cell tumor (SLCT). The investigators also tabulated 19 previously reported cases of familial SLCT, or SLCT associated with MNG, and the mean age of the 15 patients with available information was 29 years (range 14–57 years). However, it should be noted that mutation status was not established in these additional cases. Slade and colleagues[17] identified germline DICER1 mutations in 3 of 6 patients with

ovarian SLCT and in 1 patient with an unclassified SCST. The 3 patients with SLCT had bilateral tumors with the first tumor presenting at 12 years in 2 patients and at 17 years in the third. More recently, 2 studies have demonstrated somatic DICER1 mutations in approximately 60% of patients with SLCT[13,18]; 4 patients included in the study by Heravi-Moussavi and colleagues,[13] 3 of whom had been included in prior studies, also had germline mutations.[16,19–21] Finally, germline mutations were identified in 9 (56%) of 16 patients with SLCT entered in the International Ovarian and Testicular Stromal Tumor Registry.[22] The mean age of patients with SLCT (including 6 additional cases without mutation analysis) was 17 years (range 3–30 years). Germline DICER1 mutations were also recorded in 1 of 12 patients with juvenile granulosa cell tumor (JGCT) and in the single patient with gynandroblastoma.[22]

As discussed in greater detail later in this article, cERMS is also a recognized component of the DICER1 syndrome,[21] and 7 patients with both SLCT and cERMS have been reported.[23–27] A germline DICER1 mutation would seem likely in this clinical scenario, although only one of these patients subsequently had confirmed genetic analysis.[28] The mean age at presentation of SLCT was 18 years (range 13–27 years) and at least 4 of the patients presented with androgenic symptoms.[24–27]

The aforementioned studies were mainly focused on the genetic aspects and/or the neoplastic and hyperplastic associations of the DICER1 syndrome and therefore included limited information on ovarian tumor pathology. However, more detailed clinicopathologic data have been presented recently in one small case series and in additional case reports.[29–33] The mean age of these cases was 16 years (range 10–28 years) and most patients presented with a pelvic mass or with androgenic symptoms. When recorded, the tumor dimensions ranged from 35 mm to 300 mm and the macroscopic appearances were usually described as predominantly solid with a variable cystic component (Fig. 1). Two tumors were stage II,[29,33] but otherwise all documented cases were confined to the ovary at presentation (stage I). Therefore, the limited currently available data suggest that ovarian SLCT arising in patients with likely germline DICER1 mutations occur at a younger age than sporadic neoplasms, with most presenting in the second decade.[15,16,22] Occasional tumors are also bilateral, a characteristic feature of hereditary neoplastic syndromes in general, and otherwise a rare occurrence in SLCT.[34,35] However, in most individual cases, the clinical and macroscopic features would not allow distinction

> **Key Features**
> OF OVARIAN SEX CORD–STROMAL
> TUMORS IN THE DICER1 SYNDROME
>
> - Moderately differentiated Sertoli-Leydig cell tumors (SLCTs) are most common
>
> - Juvenile granulosa cell tumor (JGCT), gynandroblastoma, and unclassified sex cord–stromal tumors (SCSTs) are also described
>
> - Presentation with pelvic mass or androgenic symptoms, usually in the second decade
>
> - Most tumors are stage I and occasional cases are bilateral
>
> - Some tumors show mixed sertoliform, (juvenile) granulosa cell tumor, and/or unclassified appearances
>
> - Heterologous elements may be more common than in sporadic SLCT and can be the dominant component
>
> - Occasional cases have retiform elements

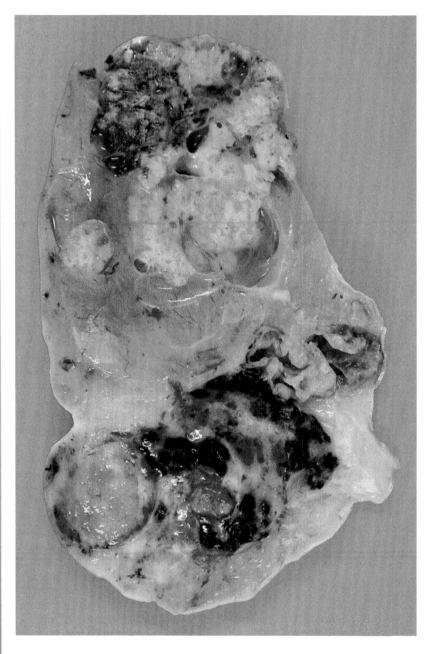

Fig. 1. Macroscopic appearance of SLCT in DICER1 syndrome. There are focally hemorrhagic pale and yellow solid tumor nodules separated by myxoid and edematous stroma.

between syndromic and sporadic SLCT unless there was a personal or family history indicative of a tumor predisposition syndrome.

HISTOLOGIC FEATURES

A recent study documented the histologic features of ovarian SCST arising in 4 patients with likely or confirmed germline *DICER1* mutations, including 3 patients from one family.[29] All tumors were classified ultimately as SLCT but 3 had distinctly varied morphologic appearances with mixed sertoliform, JGCT-like, and indeterminate or unclassified components (Figs. 2 and 3). Not surprisingly, these tumors presented diagnostic difficulty and one case was initially interpreted to be a granulosa cell tumor before expert review. The remaining tumor in this small series mainly demonstrated heterologous mucinous epithelial and neuroendocrine (carcinoid) elements. A minor heterologous component of mucinous glands and hepatoid elements was present in one other case and this also showed focal retiform appearances (Fig. 4).

Fig. 2. Low magnification showing nodular tumor appearances. (*A*) Expansile nodule (*center-right*) is composed of branching sex cord structures. (*B*) Some nodules show folliclelike spaces reminiscent of JGCT (hematoxylin-eosin [H&E], magnification × 20).

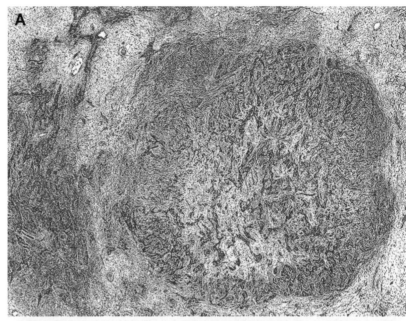

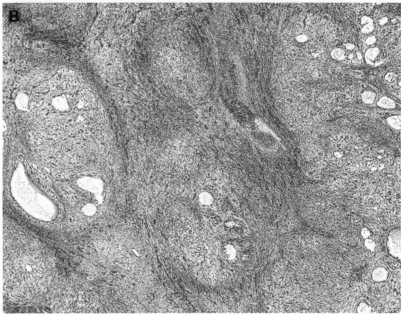

The present investigators have reviewed an additional ovarian SCST arising in a patient with an established constitutional *DICER1* mutation.[36] The tumor was reported initially to be an adult-type granulosa cell tumor, but on review was favored to be a moderately differentiated (intermediate grade) SLCT with a minor heterologous hepatoid component. Two additional tumors that were documented initially in case reports,[19,20] and subsequently reviewed in the aforementioned study of ovarian SCST and familial MNG,[16] were also moderately differentiated SLCT. None of these additional cases were recorded to show JGCT-like or retiform elements.

There are few further detailed histologic descriptions of ovarian SCST in patients with likely germline *DICER1* mutations. However, although most tumors have been interpreted to be SLCT there are also reports of JGCT, gynandroblastoma, and unclassified SCST.[15,17,22] One tumor in the series of Krisemen and colleagues[27] was described as a "high-grade mixed Sertoli and granulosa cell

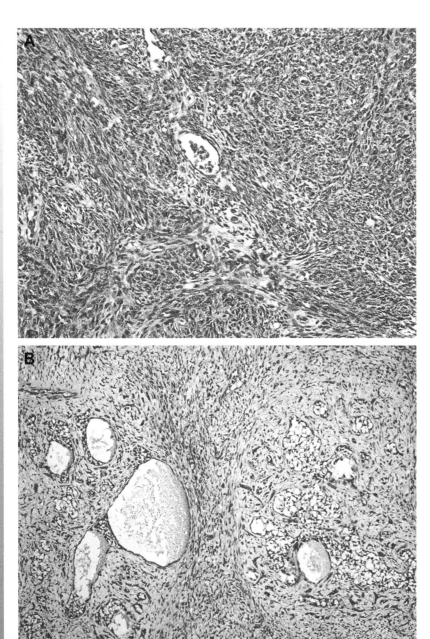

Fig. 3. Higher magnification showing variable architectural and cytologic tumor appearances. (A) Spindle cell pattern without distinct differentiation. (B) Folliclelike structures.

tumor," and Schultz and colleagues[30] commented that in their experience ovarian tumors in the DICER1 syndrome sometimes exhibited both SLCT and JGCT features. These reports, together with the findings of Oost and colleagues,[29] suggest that DICER1 syndrome–related ovarian SCST may have a tendency to exhibit heterogeneous morphologic appearances. In practice, the subclassification of such cases may depend on the relative sampled proportions of each tumor component and their interpretation by individual pathologists. As noted previously, it is pertinent that in 2 cases the initial diagnosis of granulosa cell tumor was revised to SLCT following histologic review. Regardless of classification issues, from a practical perspective, pathologists should consider the possibility of an underlying germline DICER1 mutation when encountering an ovarian SCST that is difficult to categorize or that demonstrates admixed Sertoli-Leydig and granulosa cell

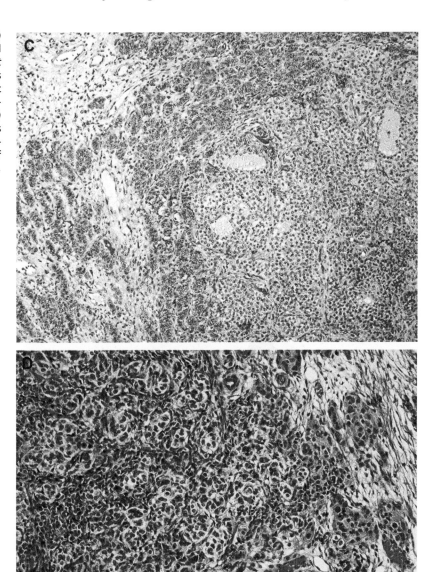

Fig. 3. (*continued*). (*C*) Trabecular and corded arrangement of cells (*left and upper*) abutting cells with more abundant cytoplasm with small folliclelike spaces (*right*). (*D*) Focal sertoliform tubules within cellular mesenchyme. Note clusters of Leydig cells (*right*) (H&E, magnification × 100).

tumor patterns. Adjunct molecular studies are likely to play an increasing role in the assessment of such diagnostically challenging SCSTs.[37–39]

DIFFERENTIAL DIAGNOSIS

With rare exceptions (discussed later in this article) ovarian neoplasms arising in the DICER1 syndrome are SCST. In most cases, the classification of these tumors as SCST will be straightforward on routine histologic examination but the diagnosis can be supported by appropriate immunohistochemical analysis if necessary.[40] However, it should be noted that currently available antibodies label most SCSTs, albeit in variable proportion, and therefore usually they will not help to subclassify those tumors that show a mixed or ambiguous sex cord–stromal phenotype.[29] The potential diagnostic role of DICER1 immunohistochemistry in this context is uncertain because most ovarian neoplasms demonstrate retained DICER1 protein

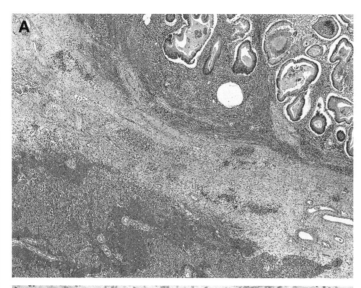

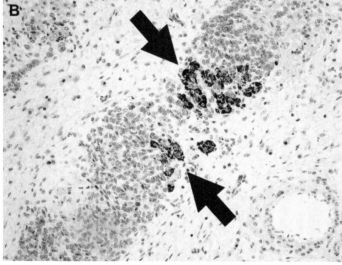

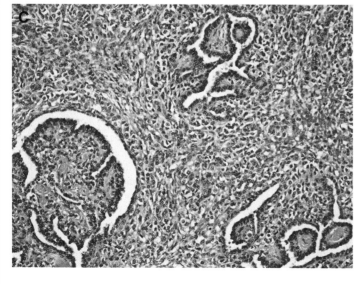

Fig. 4. (A) Glands lined by heterologous mucinous epithelium are present at upper right (H&E, magnification × 40). (B) Immunostaining for hepatocyte specific antigen highlights foci of hepatoid differentiation (arrows, immunohistochemistry, magnification × 200). (C) Focal retiform component is present (H&E, magnification × 200).

expression, whereas variable loss of staining has been noted in other tumors and in MNG.[13,16,21]

One specific diagnostic difficulty worthy of consideration is presented by SLCTs with heterologous elements, because occasionally these can predominate and thus mask the underlying sex cord–stromal neoplasm (Fig. 5).[41,42] Heterologous elements, which are present in approximately 20% of SLCTs,[34] have been described in several confirmed or likely DICER1 syndrome–associated cases and they may be more common in this condition.[15,25,28,29,33,43,44] Mucinous epithelial (enteric), neuroendocrine, and hepatoid elements have been recorded, as well as sarcomatous stromal elements. One unique tumor demonstrated a heterologous endometrioidlike yolk sac component.[26] It is not clear at present whether SLCTs in the DICER1 syndrome are more likely to show retiform elements, but these have been noted in occasional cases.[15,29,45] However, Conlon and colleagues[18] found no association between the presence of heterologous or retiform elements

Fig. 5. (*A*) SLCT with dominant epithelial and neuroendocrine (carcinoid) differentiation (*left and center*). The minor sex cord component is limited to the subcapsular stroma (*arrow*) and is indistinct at scanning power (H&E, magnification × 20). (*B*) Higher magnification showing Sertoli cell tubules and surrounding Leydig cells (H&E, magnification × 200).

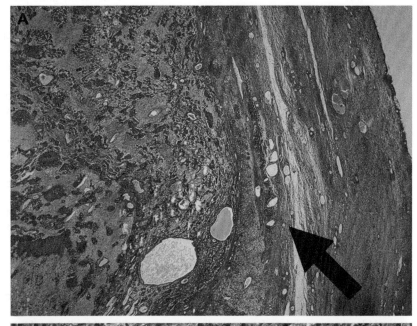

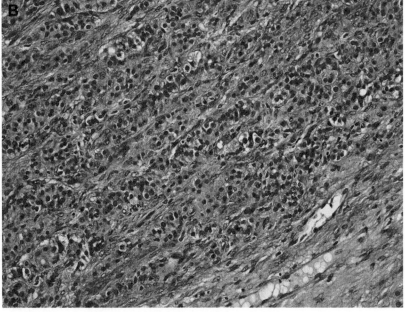

and the presence of somatic *DICER1* mutations in SLCT.

PROGNOSIS

Ovarian SCSTs, including SLCT, have a generally favorable prognosis. Moderately differentiated SLCTs, which appear to comprise most of DICER1 syndrome–related cases, have a recurrence risk of approximately 10%, although cases with heterologous mesenchymal components are considered to be more aggressive clinically.[34] Interestingly, a recent small study suggested that SLCTs with somatic *DICER1* mutations may have a higher relapse rate than mutation-negative tumors.[39] However, although recurrences have been documented in patients with likely germline *DICER1* mutations,[15,22,24,27,43] at present there are insufficient data to determine whether such cases carry a higher risk of metastases than sporadic SLCTs.

CERVICAL EMBRYONAL RHABDOMYOSARCOMA

BACKGROUND AND CLINICAL FEATURES

Key features of cERMS in the DICER syndrome are summarized in the "Key Features" box. Rhabdomyosarcoma is the most common type of cervical sarcoma but is still very rare with approximately 150 cases reported.[46] Most cases have polypoid appearances (macroscopically sarcoma botryoides, in older parlance) and present with vaginal bleeding; much less frequently the tumors form an infiltrating mass. Most cases are confined to the cervix at diagnosis and some are amenable to local excisional procedures, with or without adjuvant therapies. Unusually for rhabdomyosarcoma, approximately a third of cases present in patients older than 20 years.[23,47] Although ERMS is one of the more common sarcomas in the pediatric age group, these tumors typically present in the head and neck or around the urogenital tract (vagina, prostate, and bladder), whereas rhabdomyosarcomas at other sites presenting in older children and adults are typically the more aggressive pleomorphic and alveolar tumor subtypes. Therefore, and as discussed later in this article, cERMS is an unusual tumor in several respects, with different presentation, histologic appearance, and prognosis to the more common ERMS occurring in childhood. These differences, and their underlying genetic basis, may separate these tumors from other ERMS, at least in a significant subset of cases.

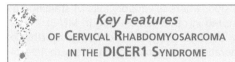

> **Key Features**
> OF CERVICAL RHABDOMYOSARCOMA
> IN THE **DICER1** SYNDROME
>
> - Presentation in older age group than typical ERMS, usually as a polypoid lesion
> - Varied histologic appearance from bland to pleomorphic and therefore wide potential differential diagnosis
> - Heterologous differentiation (cartilage) is common
> - Generally good prognosis

Because institutional-based series show that a significant minority of patients (approximately 20%) with cERMS also have additional DICER1-associated tumors,[27] the diagnosis should prompt consideration of the DICER1 syndrome, including a careful review of the patient's personal and family history with genetic studies if appropriate. It is also noteworthy that although those patients with either proven germline *DICER1* mutations or DICER1-associated cERMS reported in the literature are relatively young (<25 years), occasional cases arise in older women.[48] Therefore, older age is not a reliable criterion for excluding DICER1 syndrome in patients presenting with cERMS.

HISTOLOGIC FEATURES

Histologically, cERMS often have central myxoid stroma with a cellular cambium layer that can be difficult to discern if the lesion is ulcerated (Fig. 6). Stromal hemorrhage may also mask the presence of the diagnostic hypercellular areas.[47] The tumor cells often do not show cross striations but immunohistochemistry will show positivity for myogenin and myoD1 (often patchy, as is typical for ERMS) and focal desmin expression; however, some tumors show extensive rhabdomyoblastic differentiation, and others are more cellular and obviously malignant (Fig. 7). The tumor cells may show larger nuclei than is typical for a small round blue cell tumor of childhood and small nucleoli may be present. Fibroblastic, stellate, and myxoid foci are common, and these may have a less obviously malignant appearance. The tumor can incorporate benign glands and this can lead to the differential diagnosis of a mixed epithelial and mesenchymal tumor. Heterologous cartilaginous differentiation, including the presence of well-differentiated cartilage nodules, is frequently seen conferring an appearance similar to PPB.[24] Another feature shared with PPB, and otherwise uncommon in

Fig. 6. (*A*) Polypoid mucosa showing mainly bland myxoid stroma with small clusters of atypical spindle cells (*arrows*, H&E, magnification × 40). (*B*) Higher magnification showing cell cluster and subtle cambium layer with condensation of cells in the subepithelial stroma (H&E, magnification × 200).

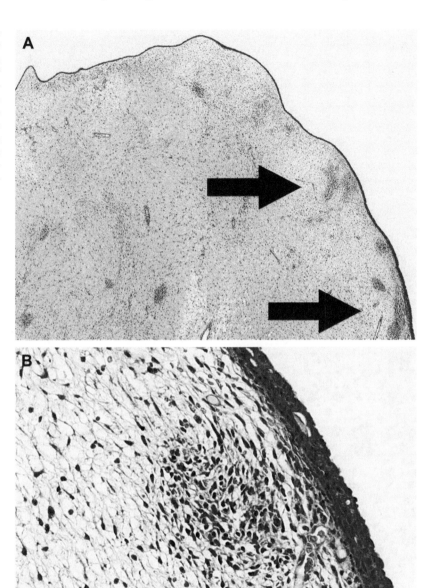

childhood rhabdomyosarcoma, is the presence of pleomorphic or anaplastic rhabdomyoblasts (see Fig. 7).[49] Less commonly, cERMS includes other elements, such as primitive neuroectodermal tissue, and occasional cases have been described as undifferentiated rhabdomyosarcoma.[24]

DIFFERENTIAL DIAGNOSIS

As a result of the variable histology of cERMS, the tumor has a potentially wide differential diagnosis.

Those cases with deceptively bland appearances and an indistinct cambium layer may mimic a benign cervical polyp, a difficultly compounded by the expression of myogenin in occasional fibroepithelial polyps.[50] The entrapped glandular epithelium surrounded by cellular stroma can lead to the consideration of adenomyoma, endometriosis, or Mullerian adenosarcoma (MAS), and the latter tumor typically shows periglandular cuffing by atypical tumor cells resembling the cambium layer of ERMS.[47] Furthermore, MAS can

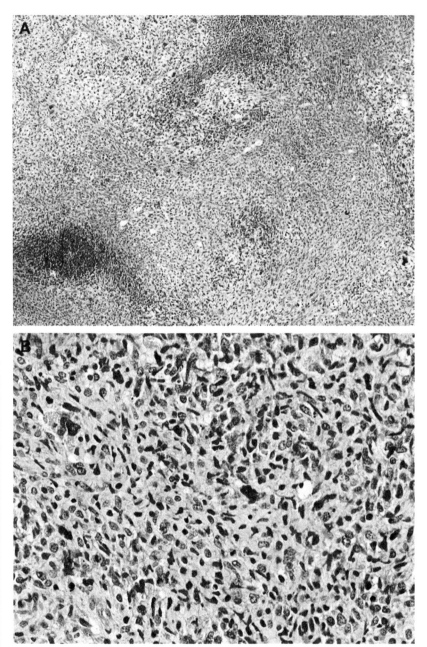

Fig. 7. (A) More cellular tumor showing obvious cytologic atypia (H&E, magnification × 100). (B) The appearances are of a pleomorphic sarcoma with no overt rhabdomyoblastic morphologic features (H&E, magnification × 400).

show heterologous rhabdomyoblastic and chondroid differentiation.[51,52]; however, MAS usually arises in the uterine body of older women and characteristically demonstrates a "phyllodeslike" architectural pattern, at least focally. Furthermore, the epithelial component of MAS has traditionally been considered neoplastic (although this has been questioned recently),[53] and often shows a range of Mullerian differentiation patterns and a nonanatomical distribution unlike the entrapped

native glands seen in cERMS. Immunohistochemistry also may be of value, as the stromal cells in MAS typically demonstrate hormone receptor expression, whereas this is uncommon in cERMS.[47]

Malignant mixed Mullerian tumor (MMMT, carcinosarcoma) also can show heterologous rhabdomyoblastic differentiation, but these tumors typically occur in postmenopausal women, much more commonly arise in the endometrium than the cervix, and by definition exhibit a malignant epithelial component. Pure mesenchymal tumors including endometrioid stromal neoplasms and smooth muscle tumors are also less likely to cause confusion with cERMS, although they rarely demonstrate skeletal muscle differentiation. These tumors also have distinctive morphologic and immunophenotypic features, and stromal neoplasms may show characteristic cytogenetic alterations.[54] Furthermore, and as with MAS and MMMT, stromal neoplasms and smooth muscle tumors much more frequently arise in the uterine corpus.

PROGNOSIS

Cervical ERMS has been described only in case studies and in a relatively small series of 11 to 14 cases in adults and children,[23,24,27] and 1 series of 20 cases in adults.[47] These reports describe a relatively favorable prognosis with more than 50% of patients being tumor-free on long-term follow-up, and only approximately 10% dying of their disease. In accord with these findings, patients with cERMS presented at lower stage and had a better 5-year prognosis than younger patients with vaginal rhabdomyosarcoma in a review of the Surveillance, Epidemiology, and End Results database.[55]

OTHER OVARIAN NEOPLASMS POSSIBLY LINKED TO DICER1 SYNDROME

There are rare reports of gynecologic sarcomas other than cERMS in patients with possible germline DICER1 mutations. Schultz and colleagues[33] reported a 10-year-old girl who developed a "poorly differentiated sarcoma with limited myogenic differentiation" in one ovary, and 4 years later developed SLCT in the contralateral ovary. Another 10-year-old patient described by Panagiotou and colleagues[45] underwent oophorectomy and partial salpingectomy for a torted retiform SLCT. She re-presented only 3 to 4 months later with ERMS in the region of the residual fallopian tube, which the investigators suggested might have been derived from a heterologous mesenchymal component of the SLCT. The mutation status of these patients was not established. Recently, de Kock and colleagues[56] reported an ovarian ERMS in a 6-year-old patient with confirmed germline DICER1 mutation. As with the case reported by Panagiotou and colleagues,[45] the investigators considered the possibility that the tumor represented sarcomatous overgrowth of an SLCT but no morphologic evidence of an underlying SCST could be demonstrated.

There is a single report of primitive neuroectodermal tumor (PNET) of the cervix (now referred to a Ewing's family tumor) in a patient with a germline DICER1 mutation,[21] and the patient reported by Panagiotou and colleagues[45] subsequently developed Ewing sarcoma of the humerus. Further studies are required to determine whether patients with germline DICER1 mutations are at increased risk of developing tumors in the PNET/Ewing sarcoma group.

Ovarian germ cell and epithelial tumors are not currently considered to be part of the DICER1 syndrome. However, cases of dysgerminoma and seminoma have been reported in genetically untested relatives of affected patients,[15] and Slade and colleagues[17] identified a possibly pathogenic missense germline mutation in 1 of 71 patients with seminoma. It is also worth noting that a minority of germ cell tumors demonstrate somatic DICER1 mutations.[13,57] However, Sabbaghian and colleagues[58] studied germline DNA from 43 familial testicular cancer kindred probands and no mutations were found.

It is possible that extensive heterologous mucinous epithelial or neuroendocrine differentiation within an SLCT could mimic a primary ovarian mucinous neoplasm or carcinoid tumor, respectively, and this could account for occasional reports of ovarian mucinous neoplasia in patients or family members with probable DICER1 mutations.[44,59] Therefore, the possibility of a constitutional DICER1 mutation is worth considering in patients presenting with other types of gynecologic neoplasia if there is a suggestive personal or family history. Conversely, tumor review may be valuable in cases in which a germline mutation is subsequently identified and the initial histologic diagnosis does not fall within the established DICER1 spectrum.[60]

ACKNOWLEDGMENTS

The authors are most grateful to John R. Priest, MD, for comments on an earlier version of this article, and to Leanne de Kock, BTech, for important laboratory contributions to some of the work described here and for providing images of the cERMS.

REFERENCES

1. Bernstein E, Caudy AA, Hammond SM, et al. Role for a bidentate ribonuclease in the initiation step of RNA interference. Nature 2001;409:363–6.

2. Grishok A, Pasquinelli AE, Conte D, et al. Genes and mechanisms related to RNA interference regulate expression of the small temporal RNAs that control *C. elegans* developmental timing. Cell 2001;106: 23–34.

3. Hutvágner G, McLachlan J, Pasquinelli AE, et al. A cellular function for the RNA-interference enzyme Dicer in the maturation of the let-7 small temporal RNA. Science 2001;293:834–8.

4. Ketting RF, Fischer SE, Bernstein E, et al. Dicer functions in RNA interference and in synthesis of small RNA involved in developmental timing in *C. elegans.* Genes Dev 2001;15:2654–9.

5. Knight SW, Bass BL. A role for the RNase III enzyme DCR-1 in RNA interference and germ line development in *Caenorhabditis elegans.* Science 2001; 293:2269–71.

6. Foulkes WD, Priest JR, Duchaine TF. DICER1: mutations, microRNAs and mechanisms. Nat Rev Cancer 2014;14:662–72.

7. Bernstein E, Kim SY, Carmell MA, et al. Dicer is essential for mouse development. Nat Genet 2003; 35:215–7.

8. Wienholds E, Koudijs MJ, van Eeden FJ, et al. The microRNA-producing enzyme DICER1 is essential for zebrafish development. Nat Genet 2003;35: 217–8.

9. Kanellopoulou C, Muljo SA, Kung AL, et al. Dicer-deficient mouse embryonic stem cells are defective in differentiation and centromeric silencing. Genes Dev 2005;19:489–501.

10. Priest JR, Watterson J, Strong L, et al. Pleuropulmonary blastoma: a marker for familial disease. J Pediatr 1996;128:220–4.

11. Hill DA, Ivanovich J, Priest JR, et al. DICER1 mutations in familial pleuropulmonary blastoma. Science 2009;325:965.

12. Foulkes WD. Inherited susceptibility to common cancers. N Engl J Med 2008;359:2143–53.

13. Heravi-Moussavi A, Anglesio MS, Cheng SW, et al. Recurrent somatic DICER1 mutations in nonepithelial ovarian cancers. N Engl J Med 2012;366: 234–42.

14. Zhang H, Kolb FA, Jaskiewicz L, et al. Single processing center models for human Dicer and bacterial RNase III. Cell 2004;118:57–68.

15. Schultz K, Pacheco M, Yang J, et al. Ovarian sex cord-stromal tumours, pleuropulmonary blastoma and DICER1 mutations: A report from the International Pleuropulmonary Blastoma Registry. Gynecol Oncol 2011;122:246–50.

16. Rio Frio T, Bahubeshi A, Kanellopoulou C, et al. DICER1 mutations in familial multinodular goiter with and without ovarian Sertoli-Leydig cell tumors. JAMA 2011;305:68–77.

17. Slade I, Bacchelli C, Davies H, et al. DICER1 syndrome: clarifying the diagnosis, clinical features and management implications of a pleiotropic tumour predisposition syndrome. J Med Genet 2011;48:273–8.

18. Conlon N, Schultheis AM, Piscuoglio S, et al. A survey of *DICER1* hotspot mutations in ovarian and testicular sex cord-stromal tumors. Mod Pathol 2015;28:1603–12.

19. O'Brien PK, Wilansky DL. Familial thyroid nodulation and arrhenoblastoma. Am J Clin Pathol 1981;75: 578–81.

20. Niedziela M. Virilizing ovarian tumor in a 14-year-old female with a prior familial multinodular goitre. Pediatr Blood Cancer 2008;51:543–5.

21. Foulkes WD, Bahubeshi A, Hamel N, et al. Extending the phenotypes associated with DICER1 mutations. Hum Mut 2011;32:1381–4.

22. Schultz KAP, Harris A, Doros L, et al. Clinical and genetic aspects of ovarian tumors: report from the international ovarian and testicular stromal tumor registry. J Clin Oncol 2014;32(15S):5520.

23. Daya DA, Scully RE. Sarcoma botryoides of the uterine cervix in young women: a clinicopathological study of 13 cases. Gynecol Oncol 1988;29: 290–304.

24. Dehner LP, Jarzembowski JA, Hill DA. Embryonal rhabdomyosarcoma of the uterine cervix: a report of 14 cases and a discussion of its unusual clinicopathologic associations. Mod Pathol 2012;25: 602–14.

25. McLean GE, Kurian S, Walter N, et al. Cervical embryonal rhabdomyosarcoma and ovarian Sertoli-Leydig cell tumour: a more than coincidental association of two rare neoplasms? J Clin Pathol 2007;60: 326–8.

26. Golbang P, Khan A, Scurry J, et al. Cervical sarcoma botryoides and ovarian Sertoli-Leydig cell tumor. Gynecol Oncol 1977;67:102–6.

27. Krisemen ML, Wang W-L, Sullinger J, et al. Rhabdomyosarcoma of the cervix in adult women and younger patients. Gynecol Oncol 2012;126:351–6.

28. Tomiak E, de Kock L, Grynspan D, et al. DICER1 mutations in an adolescent with cervical embryonal rhabdomyosarcoma (cERMS). Pediatr Blood Cancer 2014;61:568–9.

29. Oost EE, Charles A, Choong CC, et al. Ovarian sex cord-stromal tumors in patients with probable or confirmed germline DICER1 mutations. Int J Gynecol Pathol 2015;34:266–74.

30. Schultz KA, Yang J, Doros L, et al. DICER1-pleuropulmonary blastoma familial tumor predisposition syndrome: a unique constellation of neoplastic conditions. Pathol Case Rev 2014;19:90–100.

31. Wu Y, Chen D, Li Y, et al. DICER1 mutations in a patient with an ovarian Sertoli-Leydig tumor, well-differentiated fetal adenocarcinoma of the lung, and familial multinodular goiter. Eur J Med Genet 2014;57:621–5.

32. Rossing M, Gerdes A-M, Juul A, et al. A novel DICER1 mutation identified in a female with ovarian Sertoli-Leydig cell tumor and multinodular goiter: a case report. J Med Case Rep 2014;8:112.

33. Schultz KAP, Harris A, Messinger Y, et al. Ovarian tumors related to intronic mutations in DICER1: a report from the international ovarian and testicular stromal tumor registry. Fam Cancer 2016;15(1):105–10.

34. Young RH, Scully RE. Ovarian Sertoli–Leydig cell tumors. A clinicopathologic analysis of 207 cases. Am J Surg Pathol 1985;9:543–69.

35. Rutter MM, Jha P, Schultz KAP, et al. DICER1 mutations and differentiated thyroid carcinoma: evidence of a direct association. J Clin Endocrinol Metab 2016;101(1):1–5.

36. Wu MK, de Kock L, Conwell LS, et al. Functional characterization of multiple DICER1 mutations in an adolescent. Endocr Relat Cancer 2016;23(2):L1–5.

37. Kommoss S, Gilks CB, Penzel R, et al. A current perspective on the pathological assessment of FOXL2 in adult-type granulosa cell tumours of the ovary. Histopathology 2014;64:380–8.

38. Stewart CJR, Alexiadis M, Crook M, et al. An immunohistochemical and molecular analysis of problematic and unclassified ovarian sex cord-stromal tumors. Hum Pathol 2013;44:2774–81.

39. Goulvent T, Ray-Coquard I, Borel S, et al. DICER1 and FOXL2 mutations in ovarian sex cord-stromal tumours: a GINECO Group study. Histopathology 2016;68(2):279–85.

40. Rabban JT, Zaloudek CJ. A practical approach to immunohistochemical diagnosis of ovarian germ cell tumours and sex cord-stromal tumours. Histopathology 2013;62:71–88.

41. Wilkinson N, Osborn S, Young RH. Sex cord-stromal tumours of the ovary: a review highlighting recent advances. Diagn Histopathol 2008;14:389–400.

42. Liang L, Menzin A, Lovecchio JL, et al. Ovarian Sertoli-Leydig cell tumor with predominant heterologous mucinous differentiation and foci of hepatocytic differentiation: case report and review of the literature. Ann Clin Lab Sci 2015;45:348–51.

43. Benfield GF, Tapper-Jones L, Stout TV. Androblastoma and raised serum alpha-fetoprotein with familial multinodular goitre. Br J Obstet Gynaecol 1982;89:323–6.

44. Goldstein DP, Lamb EJ. Arrhenoblastoma in first cousins. Report of 2 cases. Obstet Gynecol 1970; 35:444–50.

45. Panagiotou JP, Polychronopoulou S, Sofou K, et al. Second and third malignant solid tumor in a girl with ovarian Sertoli-Leydig tumor. Pediatr Blood Cancer 2006;46:654–6.

46. Fadare O. Uncommon sarcomas of the uterine cervix: a review of selected entities. Diagn Pathol 2006;1:30.

47. Li RF, Gupta M, McCluggage WG, et al. Embryonal rhabdomyosarcoma (botryoid type) of the uterine corpus and cervix in adult women: report of a case series and review of the literature. Am J Surg Pathol 2013;37:344–55.

48. de Kock L, Boshari T, Martinelli F, et al. Adult-onset cervical embryonal rhabdomyosarcoma and DICER1 mutations. J Low Genit Tract Dis 2016;20:e8–10.

49. Houghton JP, McCluggage WG. Embryonal rhabdomyosarcoma of the cervix with focal pleomorphic areas. J Clin Pathol 2007;60:88–9.

50. McCluggage WG, Longacre TA, Fisher C. Myogenin expression in vulvovaginal spindle cell lesions: analysis of a series of cases with an emphasis on diagnostic pitfalls. Histopathology 2013;63:545–50.

51. Clement PB, Scully RE. Mullerian adenosarcoma of the uterus: a clinicopathologic analysis of 100 cases with a review of the literature. Hum Pathol 1990;21: 363–81.

52. McCluggage WG. Mullerian adenosarcoma of the female genital tract. Adv Anat Pathol 2010;17:122–9.

53. Piscuoglio S, Burke KA, Ng CK, et al. Uterine adenosarcomas are mesenchymal neoplasms. J Pathol 2016;238(3):381–8.

54. Chiang S, Oliva E. Recent developments in uterine mesenchymal neoplasms. Histopathology 2013;62: 124–37.

55. Kirsch CH, Goodman M, Esiashvili N. Outcome of female pediatric patients diagnosed with genital tract rhabdomyosarcoma based on analysis of cases registered in SEER database between 1973 and 2006. Am J Clin Oncol 2014;37:47–50.

56. de Kock L, Druker H, Weber E, et al. Ovarian embryonal rhabdomyosarcoma is a rare manifestation of the DICER1 syndrome. Hum Pathol 2015; 46:917–22.

57. Witkowski L, Mattina J, Schonberger S, et al. DICER1 hotspot mutations in non-epithelial gonadal tumours. Br J Cancer 2013;109:2744–50.

58. Sabbaghian N, Bahubeshi A, Shuen AY, et al. Germline DICER1 mutations do not make a major contribution to the etiology of familial testicular germ cell tumours. BMC Res Notes 2013;6:127.

59. Jensen RD, Norris HJ, Fraumeni JF. Familial arrhenoblastoma and thyroid adenoma. Cancer 1974;33: 218–23.

60. Cross SF, Arbuckle S, Priest JR, et al. Familial pleuropulmonary blastoma in Australia. Pediatr Blood Cancer 2010;55:1417–9.

Peutz-Jeghers Syndrome

Pathobiology, Pathologic Manifestations, and Suggestions for Recommending Genetic Testing in Pathology Reports

Emily E.K. Meserve, MD, MPH, Marisa R. Nucci, MD*

KEYWORDS

- Gastric-type endocervical adenocarcinoma • Minimal deviation adenocarcinoma
- Adenoma malignum • Sex cord tumor with annular tubules • Sertoli cell tumor
- *STK11/LKB1* • Tumor suppressor

Key points

- Peutz-Jeghers syndrome (PJS) is a clinical syndrome usually characterized by gastrointestinal, especially small bowel, hamartomatous polyposis and mucocutaneous melanin pigmentation.
- Germline mutations in *STK11/LKB1* are found in a majority of PJS patients. Other potential susceptibility genes have yet to be confirmed.
- Sex cord tumors with annular tubules (SCTATs) associated with PJS are usually bilateral and microscopic, in contrast to the sporadic form, which is often unilateral, large, and cystic.
- *STK11/LKB1* mutation in gastric-type endocervical adenocarcinoma (GAS) is associated with worse prognosis.
- Although rare, gynecologic pathologists can recognize PJS-associated manifestations in the female genital tract and be helpful in recommending additional genetic testing and/or counseling.

ABSTRACT

Peutz-Jeghers syndrome (PJS), in most cases, is attributed to mutation in *STK11/LKB1* and is clinically characterized by gastrointestinal hamartomatous polyposis, mucocutaneous pigmentation, and predisposition to certain neoplasms. There are currently no recommended gynecologic screening or clinical surveillance guidelines beyond those recommended for the general population; however, cervical cytology samples must be examined with a high level of suspicion for cervical adenocarcinoma. It is considered prudent to note the established association with PJS and recommend referral for genetic counseling. Complete surgical excision after a diagnosis of atypical lobular endocervical glandular hyperplasia is recommended.

OVERVIEW

This article begins with a review of the history, clinical features, and pathobiological underpinnings of PJS and continues with focused discussion of associated gynecologic neoplasms. Those discussed in detail are ovarian SCTATs, Sertoli cell tumors, and GAS, including its well-differentiated form. The clinical features, gross pathologic findings, key histologic features, common differential

Disclosure Statement: Neither author has any disclosures.
Division of Women's and Perinatal Pathology, Department of Pathology, Brigham and Women's Hospital, 75 Francis Street, Boston, MA 02115, USA
* Corresponding author.
E-mail address: mnucci@partners.org

diagnoses, and the use of immunohistochemistry are discussed for each entity. PJS is an inherited syndrome, and patients may be diagnosed early in life; therefore, recommendations for preventive screening and clinical surveillance for gynecologic tract neoplasia are also covered. Lastly, recommendations are made to guide practicing surgical pathologists regarding when it is appropriate to suggest additional genetic counseling or testing based on findings documented in a surgical pathology report.

INTRODUCTION

HISTORY OF THE DISEASE

The first comprehensive descriptions of the inherited form of PJS are credited to Drs Jan Peutz and Harold Jeghers, who both described patients with gastrointestinal hamartomatous polyps, especially in the small intestine, and mucocutaneous melanin pigmentation—the latter distinguishing PJS from previously described gastrointestinal polyposis syndromes. Although both recognized the inherited nature of the syndrome, Dr Jeghers correctly postulated an autosomal dominant inheritance pattern.[1,2]

Despite the eponymous recognition given to Peutz and Jeghers, J.R.T Connor is acknowledged to have given the first description of PJS in a brief report to the Aesculapian Society of London in 1895, in which he described 12-year-old twin girls with a unique form of mucosal pigmentation characterized as small pigmented spots "scattered over the lips (especially the lower), gums and hard palate but not the tongue."[1,3] These same twins were the subject of Sir Jonathan Hutchinson's 1896 description of the pigmentation; both girls lacked symptoms of gastrointestinal polyposis at the time of these initial reports. More than 50 years later, however, a report of clinical follow-up documented that 1 twin had died at age 20 due to complications of intussusception, presumably resulting from intestinal polyposis, although this was not pathologically confirmed. The other twin died of breast cancer at age 52 without available data regarding gastrointestinal symptoms.[4]

In 1956, a case series and literature review of PJS patients was published wherein the investigators performed the first detailed microscopic examination of polyps from the small bowel, colon, and stomach and morphologically distinguished and correctly classified them as hamartomatous based on the presence of histologically unremarkable epithelium and bands of smooth muscle in stroma. This group further distinguished PJS from other adenomatous familial polyposis syndromes by noting the very low rate of gastrointestinal malignancy in PJS and hypothesized that epithelium associated with the characteristic arborizing smooth muscle fibers may have been misinterpreted in prior reports as myoinvasive tumor (Fig. 1). Based on the approximately 75 published cases at the time, the investigators documented equal gender and racial distribution and further expanded the known distribution of pigmentation to include involvement of the eyelids, hard palate, tongue, rectal mucosa, and peritoneum.[2] These investigators also postulated de novo mutation occurring in patients without affected family members.[5]

Subsequently, the clinical manifestations of PJS were quickly expanded to include polyps arising in additional anatomic sites, including the esophagus, bladder, ureter, renal pelvis, bronchus, and nasal passages, and by 1957 a high rate of ovarian cysts and tumors had been noted.[6,7] In 1970, Scully[8] published the original description of a novel ovarian neoplasm, termed SCTATs, based on a series of 13 cases, including 6 from PJS patients, and reported the broad spectrum of ovarian neoplasia observed in PJS patients, including, up to that point, cystadenoma, granulosa cell tumor, dysgerminoma, and carcinosarcoma. Sertoli cell tumor of the ovary and well-differentiated endocervical adenocarcinoma were later added to the list of gynecologic neoplasms associated with PJS.[9–13]

The clinical description of PJS has changed little in the past 25 years. During this time period, however, major contributions have occurred in understanding the genetic causes and molecular pathogenesis of PJS, discussed in detail later.

CLINICAL FEATURES

PJS occurs in sporadic and in autosomal dominant inherited forms and in both can show impressive heterogeneity in clinical manifestations. Mucocutaneous pigmentation occurs in approximately 95% of PJS patients and is characterized by typically small (1–5 mm) pigmented macules commonly distributed around the mouth, eyes, nostrils, and perianal area and less often on the fingers, toes, hands, and feet.[3,14] Skin pigmentation may be present at birth or appear during early infancy. In some cases, it may fade with age; however, pigmentation of the buccal mucosa can persist. These macules generally cause no other symptoms and have not been associated with neoplastic transformation.[3] In the gastrointestinal tract, hamartomatous polyps tends to appear early in life, most commonly in the small intestine, especially the jejunum, followed by colon, rectum, and,

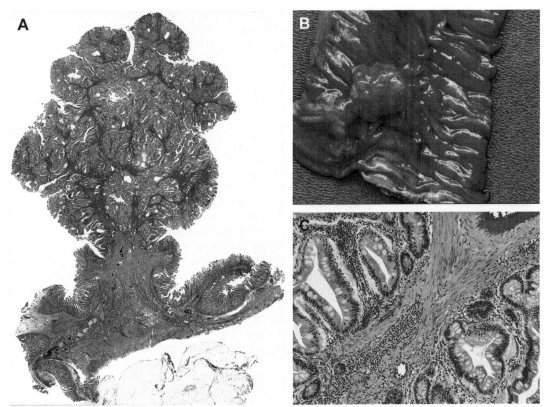

Fig. 1. PJS-associated polyp of the small intestine. (*A*) Whole-slide scan and (*B*) gross image demonstrating a large, pedunculated polyp with arborizing bands of myomatous stroma. (*C*) Higher-power magnification demonstrates a lack of adenomatous epithelium; instead, lining epithelium is similar to non-neoplastic epithelium of the small intestine (H&E, 20×).

lastly, stomach. Polyps of the small and large intestine are usually large and pedunculated, often leading to recurrent episodes of intussuception and abdominal pain. In contrast, those in the stomach tend to be sessile. Patients also may experience gastrointestinal bleeding, leading to iron deficiency anemia.[3] Polyps may occur in other anatomic sites, including nasal passages, bronchi, biliary tract, ureter, and bladder.[3,15] PJS is also associated with an increased risk of neoplasia–notably breast, gastrointestinal, endocervical, and, less commonly, thyroid, lung, and pancreatic cancers.[15] Male patients with PJS may rarely develop unique tumors of the testis, called large cell calcifying Sertoli cell tumor (alternatively, testicular tumors resembling SCTAT), and may also develop gynecomastia and advanced bone age early in life. Gynecologic findings associated with PJS include mucinous metaplasia of the fallopian tube, endocervical adenocarcinoma, and ovarian tumors, such as cystic mucinous neoplasms, SCTAT, and Sertoli cell tumors.[3]

PATHOBIOLOGICAL UNDERPINNINGS

Initial studies in the late 1990s demonstrated linkage between PJS and a susceptibility locus at chromosome 19p13.3.[16] In this candidate region, a novel serine-threonine kinase (serine/threonine kinase 11/liver kinase B1, *STK11/LKB1*), believed to function as a tumor suppressor gene, was identified and found mutated in the germline of approximately half of PJS patients.[17] *STK11/LKB1* is 23 kilobases with 9 coding exons and 1 noncoding exon. A variety of deletion, insertion, inversion, and nonsense mutations have been described in nearly every coding exon, predominantly in exons 1, 5, 6, and 7.[3,18] Many of the described mutations lead to truncated protein with incomplete catalytic domains predicted to disrupt kinase activity.[3,17] Approximately 75% of PJS patients are estimated to have germline mutation in *STK11/LKB1*.[2]

The mechanisms by which *STK11/LKB1* mutation results in hamartomatous polyps, mucocutaneous melanin pigmentation, and neoplasia are complex. In the inherited form of PJS, loss of heterozygosity is believed the initiating event in neoplasia; however, studies of hamartomatous polyp formation in the presence of a heterozygous germline mutation suggest that biallelic inactivation is not required for hamartoma formation.[19,20]

Currently, it is believed that STK11/LKB1 is regulated by AMPK via mammalian target of rapamycin (mTOR) signaling and is thought to subsequently phosphorylate at least 14 downstream kinases.[20,21] In terms of tumor suppressor function, an important substrate of STK11/LKB1 is AMPK, which has a master regulatory role in cellular metabolism by increasing catabolic processes in response to hypoxia or glucose deprivation.[20,22] Additionally, multiple other cellular functions have been attributed to STK11/LKB1, including cell proliferation, cellular polarity, cellular migration, DNA damage response, and cellular differentiation, possibly through regulatory effects on AMPK, transforming growth factor β, and/or Wnt signaling pathways.[20,23]

STK11/LKB1 mutations are rarely found in sporadic or PJS-associated gastrointestinal and breast cancers but are found in some sporadic lung and endocervical adenocarcinomas.[24–29] It has also been shown that STK11/LKB1 is not uniquely involved in cases of sporadic SCTAT, but loss of heterozygosity at 19p13.3 is seen in these tumors, suggesting the possibility of an alternative albeit closely located mutated gene.[30] Investigators have demonstrated STK11/LKB1 mutation in approximately 50% of sporadic mucinous well-differentiated endocervical adenocarcinomas and show that the presence of a STK11/LKB1 mutation among sporadic cases is associated with significantly poorer prognosis.[29]

Early in the investigation of the gene responsible for PJS, a second potential susceptibility locus was identified on 19q13.4.[31] Subsequent studies investigating candidate genes in this region as well as STK11/LKB1-interacting protein have failed to identify mutations within PJS families without STK11/LKB1 mutations.[32,33] Additional studies focusing on mutation analysis of proteins known to interact with STK11/LKB1 have also failed to identify mutations.[34,35]

In summary, mutation in STK11/LKB1 is associated with most cases of inherited PJS. STK11/LKB1 may function as a haploinsufficient tumor suppressor gene in the pathogenesis of gastrointestinal hamartomatous polyps. The mechanisms by which mutations in STK11/LKB1 induce neoplasia are complex and not fully elucidated. STK11/LKB1 mutation does not seem to play a major role in PJS-associated gastrointestinal or breast cancers but is detected in sporadic and PJS-associated endocervical adenocarcinomas.

It remains to be determined whether a second susceptibility gene will be confirmed in PJS patients without STK11/LKB1 mutation.

GYNECOLOGIC TUMORS IN PEUTZ-JEGHERS SYNDROME

SEX CORD TUMOR WITH ANNULAR TUBULES

Brief Introduction

The SCTAT was initially described by Dr. Scully based on morphologic observations of a neoplasm that resembled primitive sex cords with cytomorphology of granulosa cells but an architectural pattern more characteristic of Sertoli cell tumors.[8] Although histogenesis of SCTAT remains controversial, more than 100 cases have subsequently been reported in the literature, with approximately one-third associated with PJS.[36] When associated with PJS, tumors typically arise in young adulthood, and patients may present with menstrual irregularity and/or hyperestrogenism.[13] SCTATs are identified in almost all women with PJS when the ovaries are microscopically examined; however, these are nearly all incidental findings due to small tumor size and almost always have benign clinical course.[37–39] In contrast, patients with SCTAT unassociated with PJS present over a wider age range from childhood to postmenopause (average 36 years) but often also with menstrual irregularities.[13] Among sporadic cases, STK11/LKB1 mutations are usually not identified, and 15% to 20% may have clinically malignant behavior.[13,40] Based on bilaterality, multifocality, and observations of similar tumors in the testis, some investigators have proposed that in PJS, SCTAT represents a hamartoma rather than a neoplasm.[3]

Gross Features

When associated with PJS, SCTATs are often small to microscopic tumors (Fig. 2A). In fewer than 30% of cases, tumors are grossly apparent as single or multiple small nodules, resulting in minimal ovarian enlargement (typically <3 cm), occasionally with a yellow cut surface. Tumors tend to be bilateral and multifocal and may be associated with calcification. Concurrent ovarian cysts or other ovarian tumors may also be identified. A prior case of malignant SCTAT in a PJS patient demonstrated large bilateral tumors with bilateral pelvic lymph node metastases.[37]

When sporadic, SCTATs are usually large (up to 20 cm), unilateral, and composed of firm nodular or cystic tissue that may be yellow to tan/pink (see Fig. 2C, D). Sporadic SCTATs are also more likely to show regions of hemorrhage and necrosis.

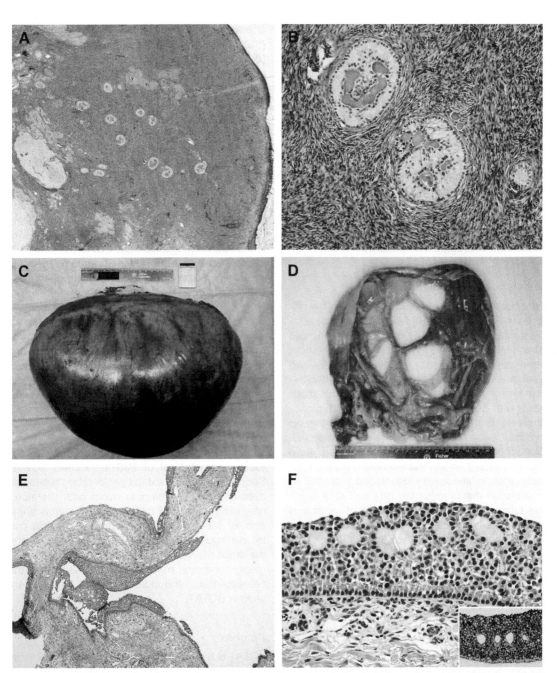

Fig. 2. SCTAT. (*A*) SCTATs associated with PJS are often bilateral, multifocal, and usually incidental findings (H&E, 2×). (*B*) Simple and complex tubular architecture within tumor nests is seen in PJS-associated and sporadic SCTATs. These nests demonstrate the classic antipodal nuclear arrangement wherein nuclei are oriented at the periphery of the nests and around the basement membrane material (H&E, 20×). (*C*) Sporadic SCTATs are more commonly large, unilateral tumors, (*D*) which are often cystic. (*E*) In cystic SCTATs, the cystic spaces are lined by epithelium that shows similar tubular architecture (H&E, 2×) with (*F*) nuclei arranged around tubules at the base of the epithelium (H&E, 40×). In both forms of SCTAT, in keeping with sex cord origin, the epithelium stains positively for inhibin (*inset*, 40×).

Microscopic Features

Both PJS-associated and sporadic SCTATs show similar microscopic features. The tumors are composed of sharply circumscribed rounded nests

of cells encircling hyalinized basement membrane–like material. The nests may be either simple, with a single tubule around the central hyalinized core, or complex, with multiple communicating tubules around multiple hyaline cores. The nuclei of the cells within the nests are characteristically located antipodally—positioned both at the periphery of the nest and around the hyaline mass(es) (see Fig. 2B, E, F). When present, calcifications typically occupy the site of the hyaline masses. Cytologically, cells within the nests show round to slightly irregular nuclei with minimal pleomorphism and small, single nucleoli, abundant, pale cytoplasm and with absent to very rare mitoses.[8,13] Variant histologic patterns have been reported, including sertoliform tubules, endometrioid areas, and foci of granulosa cell-like differentiation.[8,41–43] Reported mitotic rates, involvement of the tumor capsule, and lymphovascular space invasion are variably associated with aggressive clinical behavior.[37]

Differential Diagnosis

Whether associated with PJS or sporadic, the differential diagnosis of SCTAT includes gonadoblastoma, Sertoli cell tumor, granulosa cell tumor, sex cord–like variant of endometrioid adenocarcinoma, insular carcinoid tumor, and benign secondary follicles (Fig. 3). Gonadoblastoma may be considered in the differential diagnosis with SCTAT because both tumors typically show nests of tumor with cells arranged around hyaline basement membrane–type material. Gonadoblastomas can be distinguished from SCTATs based on several features: (1) they typically arise in abnormally developed gonads, an association that is extremely rare for SCTATs; (2) the tumor cell nests are a mixture of germ and sex cord cells, which can be confirmed by immunohistochemistry; and (3) the nuclei lack the characteristic antipodal arrangement seen in SCTATs.[44] A Sertoli cell tumor may be considered in the differential diagnosis from low-power magnification based on the appearance of tubular architecture; however, a pure Sertoli cell tumor generally lacks the complex tubular architecture seen in most SCTATs and also lacks the hyalinized basement membrane cores and antipodal nuclear arrangement. Adult-type granulosa cell tumor appears in the differential diagnosis due to overlapping cytomorphologic features and potential architectural similarity, especially the microfollicular pattern of the former wherein cells are arranged around lumens with eosinophilic material. These 2 entities can be distinguished, however, because granulosa cell tumor often demonstrates more sheet-like and large, irregular, nested architecture in contrast to the small, round, nested appearance typical of SCTAT; lacks nuclear palisading at the periphery of nests; lacks antipodal nuclear arrangement; exhibits

characteristic cytomorphology, including nuclear grooves; and shows mutation in *FOXL2*.[45] Due to shared sex cord origin, immunohistochemistry is otherwise generally not helpful in distinguishing SCTAT from a Sertoli cell tumor or granulosa cell tumor. Sex cord–like variant of endometrioid adenocarcinoma is a consideration in the differential diagnosis and can be distinguished from SCTAT based on lack of well-developed SCTAT morphology and a growth pattern in the sex cord-like areas that more typically resembles adult granulosa cell tumor, its association with a conventional endometrioid component that may show squamous differentiation, and positivity for epithelial membrane antigen (EMA) and lack of inhibin staining. Additionally, this tumor is usually associated with endometriosis and may display prominent stromal luteinization, features not typically seen in SCTAT.[46] Insular carcinoid tumor may also be considered as a differential diagnostic consideration due to its nested appearance with some tubule formation; however, the chromatin texture is more typical of neuroendocrine tumors (salt-and-pepper appearance), and cells stain positively for neuroendocrine markers (eg, synaptophysin and chromogranin) and are negative for markers of sex cord differentiation (eg, inhibin and WT1). Benign secondary follicles may be considered in the differential diagnosis, especially when they are multiple, mimicking the multifocal nature typical of PJS-associated SCTAT. Secondary follicles exhibit proliferating granulosa cells around a developing ovum and, therefore, may mimic a nest of cells in SCTAT with a single annular tubule. A benign secondary follicle can be distinguished from SCTAT based on (1) the presence of an ovum and lack of hyalinized basement membrane material and (2) the lack of the characteristic antipodal nuclear arrangement seen in SCTAT.

Diagnosis

SCTAT is typically diagnosed after oophorectomy performed for removal of an ovarian mass or is discovered as an incidental finding in an ovary removed for another indication. Gross and microscopic features are most essential for determining the diagnosis. If necessary, immunohistochemical stains, such as inhibin, calretinin, and WT1, can be used to support sex cord origin.[47] SCTAT is positive for cytokeratin but negative for EMA and germ cell markers.[48]

SCTAT has been observed in cytologic preparations on only rare occasions. A single report of fine-needle aspiration of a SCTAT describes the cytologic features as indistinguishable from those

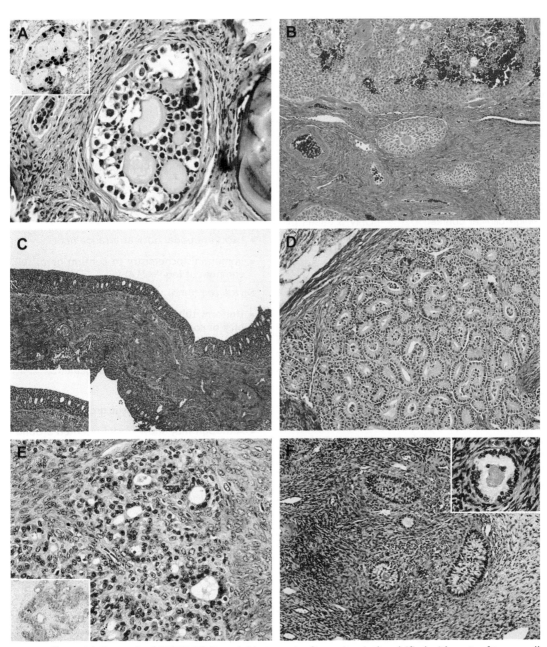

Fig. 3. Differential diagnosis of SCTAT. (*A*) Gonadoblastoma is often extensively calcified with nests of tumor cells with tubule-like structures (H&E, 40×). Tumor nests are composed of a mixture of sex cord and germ cells, which can be confirmed immunohistochemically (OCT3/4 [*inset*], 40×). (*B*) The microfollicular architecture of adult granulosa cell tumor, which sometimes may form small rounded rests of tumor cells, may mimic SCTAT (H&E, 20×). (*C*) Microfollicular adult granulosa cell tumor may also be cystic, specifically mimicking the sporadic form of SCTAT (H&E, 2×). (*inset*) In both cystic and noncystic forms of adult granulosa cell tumor, antipodal nuclear arrangement is lacking (H&E, 20×). (*D*) A pure Sertoli cell tumor showing extensive tubular architecture may resemble SCTAT but lacks the characteristic antipodal nuclear arrangement and eosinophilic basement membrane material (H&E, 20×). (*E*) Insular carcinoid may show a tubular architecture (H&E, 40×), but this tumor typically exhibits salt-and-pepper chromatin and classically shows immunoreactivity for markers of neuroendocrine differentiation (chromogranin [*inset*], 40×). (*F*) Occasionally, unusual forms of follicular differentiation may mimic SCTAT, especially when multifocal and microscopic (H&E, 20×). These follicles may also show a central eosinophilic material (*inset*) but lack well-developed antipodal nuclear arrangement (H&E, 60×).

of a granulosa cell tumor.[49] In a case report of malignant SCTAT associated with PJS, peritoneal washings concurrent to a hysterectomy demonstrated 3-D groups of cells with nuclei polarized toward the periphery of the group. Intraoperative touch preparations showed central cores of acellular hyaline material surrounded by cells that were morphologically similar to those in the peritoneal washings.[37]

Prognosis

The prognosis of PJS-associated SCTAT is very good, with nearly all reported cases having a benign clinical course.[13,42,50–52] Only 3 cases of PJS-associated malignant SCTAT exist in the literature.[37–39] In 2 cases, the patients experienced multiple tumor recurrences despite chemotherapy and radiation.[38,39] In 1 case, the patient was disease-free 28 months after diagnosis and completion of 4 cycles of chemotherapy, dose-reduced due to bone marrow toxicity.[37] In 1 case, the morphology of the recurrent tumor was predominately cords and poorly formed and solid tubular structures in myxoid to hyalinized stroma – notably lacking the typical appearance of SCTAT.[38]

At present, the malignant potential of SCTAT cannot be reliably determined by microscopic examination because usual features indicative of malignancy, such as tumor involvement of the ovarian surface, high mitotic rate, and lymphovascular space invasion, are not consistently associated with aggressive clinical behavior.[13,37–39,42,50–52] Among sporadic and PJS-associated malignant cases, early (3 months) and late (up to 20 years) recurrences have been documented and spread via lymphatics is typical, commonly involving the pelvic, para-aortic, and supraclavicular lymph nodes; spread to the pelvic peritoneum, retroperitoneum, and lung also is documented.[13,42,50–52]

Pathologic Key Features

- PJS-associated SCTAT is usually bilateral, multicentric, and microscopic whereas sporadic SCTAT is usually unilateral, large, and cystic.

- Microscopically, tumors are composed of usually small, rounded, well-circumscribed nests of cells forming simple and complex tubules with nuclei in antipodal arrangement around hyalinized basement membrane material.

- SCTAT associated with PJS almost always has a benign clinical course. Aggressive clinical behavior cannot be predicted accurately by microscopic examination.

Differential Diagnosis

Gonadoblastoma
- Typically arises in abnormally developed gonads
- Composed of a mixture of germ and sex cord cells
- Lacks antipodal nuclear arrangement
- Immunohistochemistry to confirm germ cell component (eg, SALL4)

Sertoli cell tumor
- Uniform tubular architecture without complex or coalescing tubules
- Lacks hyalinized basement membrane cores
- Lacks antipodal nuclear arrangement

Granulosa cell tumor
- Shows other characteristic growth patterns
- Although may show nuclei oriented around lumen, lacks nuclear palisading at the periphery of the well-circumscribed nests
- Mutation in *FOXL2*

Sex cord–like variant of endometrioid adenocarcinoma
- Association with endometriosis
- Lacks hyalinized basement membrane cores
- Lacks antipodal nuclear arrangement
- May display squamous or mucinous differentiation
- Positive for EMA

Insular carcinoid tumor
- Fine salt-and-pepper chromatin texture as is typical of neuroendocrine tumors
- Positive for neuroendocrine markers (eg, synaptophysin and chromogranin) and negative for markers of sex cord differentiation (eg, inhibin and WT1)

Benign secondary follicles
- Usually only single secondary follicle
- Proliferating granulosa cells around a developing ovum
- Lacks antipodal nuclear arrangement

Pitfalls

! Due to shared sex cord–stromal origin, immunohistochemical profile of SCTAT may overlap with Sertoli cell and granulosa cell tumors and is, therefore, not helpful in this diagnostic distinction.

! SCTAT may be positive for cytokeratins but is EMA negative.

OVARIAN SERTOLI CELL TUMOR

Brief Introduction

Ovarian Sertoli cell tumor was originally described by Pick in 1905 and is now classified as a subtype of pure sex cord tumors.[53,54] Most occur in women of reproductive age, but some also occur in young girls and postmenopausal women. Initial presenting symptoms are variable, in part due to patient age at presentation but can include sexual precocity, primary amenorrhea, postmenopausal bleeding, abdominal pain, and swelling. Occasionally, tumors are discovered only incidentally.[55] Symptoms are usually attributed to hyperestrinism, less commonly hyperandrogenism, and, rarely, signs and symptoms of progesterone, renin, or aldosterone excess.[41,55,56] Tumors often present at low stage and are most commonly treated with salpingo-oophorectomy with or without hysterectomy. Chemotherapy and/or radiation may be given to women with advanced-stage disease.[55]

Gross Features

Tumor size is variable (range, 0.8–30 cm), although most are usually between 4 and 12 cm.[53,55] They are typically solid but sometimes lobulated, yellow to white to tan/brown, well-circumscribed masses. Occasionally, they may be solid and cystic or predominately cystic. Necrosis and/or hemorrhage may occur.[53,55]

Microscopic Features

Sertoli cell tumors often demonstrate a diffuse to nodular growth of closely packed solid and/or hollow tubules, cords and trabeculae, or sheets of cells (**Fig. 4**A, C–E). Hollow tubules are sometimes cystically dilated, and if material is present in the lumen, it is usually eosinophilic. Trabeculae and cords may be long or short and are typically 1 to 3 cell layers thick. Rarely, retiform and alveolar-like growth patterns have been described. Pseudopapillary growth with hyalinized stroma may be appreciated.

The cells are typically cuboidal to columnar with moderate amounts of pale pink cytoplasm with round to oval, regularly shaped nuclei with inconspicuous nucleoli (see **Fig. 4**B). Moderate to severe cytologic atypia may occur. Bizarre-type cytologic atypia is rare and when encountered has been reported as more in keeping with degenerative change. Tubules may show endometrioid-like cytomorphology and, rarely, spindled, oxyphilic, or lipid-rich cells may be seen.[55] Rarely, Sertoli cell tumors may show areas with granulosa cell and SCTAT morphology. Any Leydig cell component, if present, is no more than minimal. Calcifications, tumor cell necrosis, and foci of hemorrhage may be seen; however, vascular invasion is absent. Mitotic count may be variable, but a majority have fewer than 2 mitoses per 10 high-power fields. Atypical mitotic figures are only rarely encountered. Steroidogenic factor 1 (SF-1) is typically positive (see **Fig. 4**F).

Differential Diagnosis

The differential diagnosis includes Sertoli-Leydig cell tumor (SLCT), endometrioid carcinoma, carcinoid tumor, and female adnexal tumor of probable wolffian origin (FATWO) (**Fig. 5**). SLCT is considered in the differential diagnosis because both contain tubules lined by columnar Sertoli cells; however, SLCT has a significant Leydig cell component composed of cells with abundant eosinophilic cytoplasm and centrally located round nuclei. Immature Sertoli cells often arranged in multiple architectural patterns are seen in intermediate/poorly differentiated SLCT but are absent in pure Sertoli cell tumor. Endometrioid carcinoma of the ovary is more common than Sertoli cell tumor but should be considered in the differential based on the appearance of well-formed glands lined by columnar cells with limited cytologic atypia. It is especially important to keep in mind the sex cord–like variant of endometrioid carcinoma, which may show a sertoliform pattern. Endometrioid carcinoma is often associated with endometriosis or an adenofibroma, whereas Sertoli cell tumors typically are not. Endometrioid carcinoma can also be distinguished based on (1) the presence of a conventional endometrioid component, (2) identification of intraluminal or intracytoplasmic mucin or squamous differentiation, and (3) cytokeratin and EMA positivity but inhibin and SF-1 negativity. Sertoli cell tumor and endometrioid carcinoma are typically both positive for cytokeratins; therefore, EMA and markers of sex

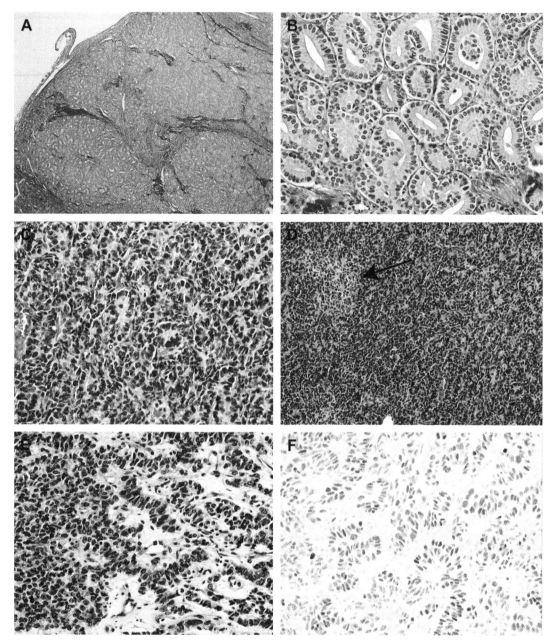

Fig. 4. Sertoli cell tumor. (*A*) Pure Sertoli cell tumor most commonly exhibits uniform tubular architecture with tubules arranged in sheets or lobules (H&E, 2×). (*B*) In well-differentiated tumors, the tubules are well-formed and lined by cytologically bland Sertoli cells (H&E, 40×). (*C*) In moderately and poorly differentiated tumors, tubules may be compressed with nuclear hyperchromasia and overlap (H&E, 20×), (*D*) may coalesce into sheets of cells with only vague tubular architecture (H&E, 2×) and necrosis (*arrow*), or (*E*) may be trabecular with single cells (H&E, 40×). (*F*) Most Sertoli tumors show immunoreactivity for SF-1 (SF-1, 40×).

cord differentiation are more reliable in this distinction. Carcinoid tumor should be also considered in the differential diagnosis of tumors with well-formed tubules lined by cuboidal to columnar epithelium. Helpful distinguishing features include the typical salt-and-pepper chromatin texture typical of neuroendocrine tumors; positive staining with neuroendocrine markers,

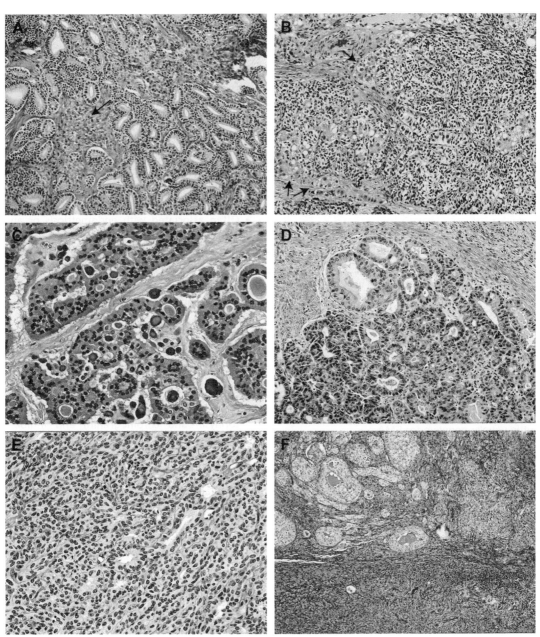

Fig. 5. Differential diagnosis of Sertoli cell tumor. (*A*) In contrast to pure Sertoli cell tumors, SLCT features a component of eosinophilic Leydig cells (*arrow*) (H&E, 10×). (*B*) In moderately and poorly differentiated SLCT, the tubular architecture of the Sertoli component may be less prominent but Leydig cells are still easily recognized (*arrow*) (H&E, 10×). (*C*) Trabecular carcinoid may also show an extensive tubular architecture but show immunoreactivity for markers of neuroendocrine differentiation (H&E, 20×). (*D*) The sex cord–like variant of endometrioid adenocarcinoma may closely mimic the tubular architecture of Sertoli cell tumor. Identifying conventional endometrioid morphology and/or mucinous and/or squamous differentiation is helpful as is EMA positivity (H&E, 20×). (*E*) FATWO usually has at least partial tubular architecture, often with compression and distortion of the tubules into sieve-like spaces, not typically seen in Sertoli cell tumor (H&E, 20×). (*F*) Hybrid sex cord–stromal tumors may show several types of differentiation, including Sertoli, granulosa, and SCTAT-like areas (H&E, 10×).

such as synaptophysin and chromogranin; and in some cases association with a teratoma or a mucinous tumor. FATWO may also exhibit a tubular architecture; however, this is often admixed with cysts with characteristic slit-like or sieve-like spaces. FATWO can be further distinguished from Sertoli cell tumor based on weak or only focal positivity for inhibin with positive staining for calretinin, CD10—typically with a luminal pattern, and cytokeratins.

Diagnosis

Patients with Sertoli cell tumor present over a broad age range with variable symptoms; most common are those associated with excess estrogen. These tumors are typically yellow, but other gross features, including size, are variable. Microscopic examination is most helpful in establishing the correct diagnosis, including identification of uniform solid and hollow tubules, cords and trabeculae, or sheets of mature Sertoli cells and lack of a significant Leydig cell component or immature Sertoli cells. Immunohistochemical markers, such as inhibin and calretinin, can be used to confirm sex cord–stromal origin. Sertoli cell tumor can show positivity for cytokeratins but is usually negative for EMA.

Prognosis

The prognosis of patients with Sertoli cell tumor is excellent, especially if it is low stage at presentation. Malignant behavior is associated with tumor size greater than 5 cm, the presence of severe nuclear atypia, or the presence of greater than 5 mitoses per 10 high-power fields.[55]

 Differential Diagnosis

Sertoli-Leydig cell tumor
- Has a significant Leydig cell component and/or immature Sertoli cells
- If intermediate or poorly differentiated, shows only a minor component of well-formed tubules with mature Sertoli cells

Endometrioid carcinoma and sex cord–like variant of endometrioid adenocarcinoma
- Often associated with endometriosis or an adenofibroma
- May have intraluminal or intracytoplasmic mucin or squamous differentiation
- Usually cytokeratin and EMA positive but inhibin and SF-1 negative

Carcinoid tumor
- May be associated with a teratoma or mucinous tumor
- Salt-and-pepper chromatin typical of neuroendocrine tumors
- Neuroendocrine marker positive (eg, synaptophysin and chromogranin) and inhibin negative

Female adnexal tumor of probable wolffian origin
- Tubular architecture often admixed with cysts with characteristic slit-like or sieve-like spaces
- Weak or focally positive for inhibin

 Pitfalls

! EMA is more helpful in the distinction between Sertoli cell tumor and endometrioid adenocarcinoma because both can be cytokeratin positive.

! Sex cord–like variant of endometrioid carcinoma can be easily confused with Sertoli cell tumor due to their shared growth pattern but is distinguished by often being associated with a conventional endometrioid component that shows squamous and/or mucinous differentiation.

Pathologic Key Features

- Patients may present over a broad age range with variable clinical symptoms but typically those associated with hyperestrinism.
- Microscopically, tumors appear as a uniform proliferation of solid or hollow tubules lined by mature Sertoli cells.
- Tumors are positive for cytokeratin but negative for EMA.

GASTRIC-TYPE ENDOCERVICAL ADENOCARCINOMA

Brief Introduction

Currently, the term *GAS* refers to endocervical adenocarcinomas that show at least partial gastric-type differentiation by histochemical or immunohistochemical studies. This diagnostic category includes well-differentiated, moderately differentiated, and poorly differentiated forms. Moderately and poorly differentiated forms of GAS are defined as tumors with any significant non–well-differentiated component or tumors composed entirely of non–well-differentiated adenocarcinoma.[54] The extremely well-differentiated form of GAS (EWDGAS) is discussed later. Historically, based on the morphologic appearance of the mucinous cytoplasm, these tumors were classified as mucinous carcinomas. They have been only recently distinguished as a unique gastric subtype of mucinous carcinoma based on identification of pyloric gland-type mucins (eg, MUC6 and HIK1083).[57,58] These tumors are characteristically unassociated with high-risk human papillomavirus (HR-HPV) infection.[59,60]

Gross Features

GAS may present as a firm and indurated mass – giving rise to so-called barrel-shaped cervical enlargement. The cut surface may be friable, hemorrhagic, mucoid or may appear cystic. Occasionally, the cervix may appear unremarkable.[61]

Microscopic Features

The moderately and poorly differentiated forms of GAS are characterized by glands invading cervical stroma typically associated with a desmoplastic stromal response. The glands, which are typically variably sized and irregularly shaped with angulated contours, extend into endocervical stroma beyond the depth of adjacent benign epithelium and beyond that typically expected for benign glandular proliferations (Fig. 6A). The glands may also fuse resulting in solid growth or a cribriform pattern. They are lined by mucinous epithelium having copious clear or pale eosinophilic cytoplasm and accentuated cell borders, resulting in a prominent "plant-like" appearance.[62] The nuclei are typically enlarged and hyperchromatic and may have eosinophilic nucleoli. Mitotic figures are usually present but the rate is variable[54,63] (see Fig. 6B, C).

Differential Diagnosis

For moderately and poorly differentiated GAS, the differential diagnosis includes usual-type endocervical adenocarcinoma; other subtypes of mucinous endocervical adenocarcinoma, including intestinal and signet ring types; and metastatic signet ring cell carcinoma (see Fig. 6D–F). Usual-type endocervical adenocarcinoma can be distinguished by a less abundant apical mucinous cytoplasm and strong p16 staining in combination with lack of markers of gastric differentiation. In equivocal cases, polymerase chain reaction (PCR) can be used to demonstrate the presence of HR-HPV, which is present in essentially all usual-type endocervical adenocarcinomas.[54] Both intestinal-type endocervical adenocarcinoma and GAS are composed of variably formed glands with or without signet ring cells that may show focal cribriform or papillary architecture and are often associated with a desmoplastic stromal response. These tumors, however, can be distinguished by cytomorphologic features because intestinal-type endocervical adenocarcinoma typically shows goblet and/or Paneth cell differentiation whereas GAS features apical, clear, or pale eosinophilic cytoplasm and distinct cell borders. In addition, by immunohistochemistry, intestinal-type endocervical adenocarcinoma is typically positive for MUC2 and p16 whereas GAS is typically positive for MUC6 and is negative or patchy positive for p16. Concordant with the p16 immunohistochemical staining patterns, HPV DNA is usually detected in intestinal-type endocervical adenocarcinoma and only rarely detected in GAS. Signet ring cell–type endocervical adenocarcinoma is rare and shows exclusively signet ring morphology. This tumor appears in the differential diagnosis with GAS because it may show gastric differentiation but, unlike GAS, is usually associated with HR-HPV.[54] Metastatic signet ring cell carcinomas from breast, lung, or stomach may mimic poorly differentiated GAS with signet ring cells. Staining with certain organ-specific markers, such as positive GATA3 staining supporting breast origin can help identify site of origin. Distinguishing metastases from the upper gastrointestinal tract from primary endocervical adenocarcinomas with gastrointestinal differentiation can be challenging due to overlapping immunohistochemical profiles.[64,65] Knowledge of a prior history of malignancy exhibiting signet ring morphology can be helpful in supporting a diagnosis of metastasis, whereas identification of an in situ component can be helpful in supporting a diagnosis of an endocervical primary.

Diagnosis

The diagnosis of GAS is primarily established based on morphologic features in combination with supportive immunohistochemistry. In straightforward cases, irregularly shaped glands deeply invade endocervical stroma with an associated desmoplastic response. The epithelium

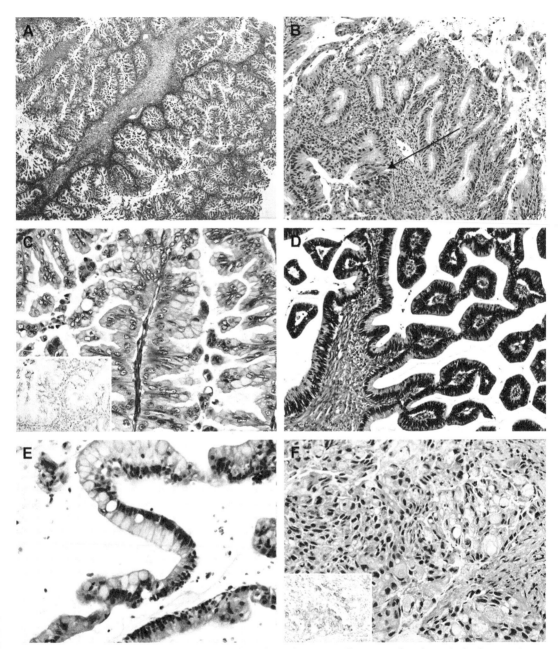

Fig. 6. GAS and differential diagnosis. (*A*) Moderately and poorly differentiated endocervical adenocarcinoma show extensive epithelial proliferation with crowded, back-to-back glands (H&E, 2×). (*B*) Cytologic atypia and mitoses are easily apparent (arrow) (H&E, 10×). (*C*) Gastric-type adenocarcinoma is characterized by voluminous pale to eosinophilic cytoplasm with distinct cell borders (H&E, 40×) and, unlike most other forms of endocervical adenocarcinoma, is usually p16 negative (*inset* (p16, 20×)). (*D*) Usual-type endocervical adenocarcinoma typically shows prominent nuclear hyperchromasia and relative mucin depletion, compared with normal endocervical mucosa. Apically located mitoses are usually easy to identify (H&E, 10×). (*E*) Intestinal adenocarcinomas can be distinguished from gastric-type adenocarcinoma based on the presence of goblet cells (H&E, 40×). (*F*) Other mucinous adenocarcinomas, including primary endocervical and metastatic signet ring cell carcinomas, may also be considered (H&E, 40×). This example shows a metastatic signet ring cell carcinoma that was CK7 (*inset*) (CK7, 40×) and TTF1 positive, in keeping with pulmonary origin.

lining these glands is cytologically atypical with frequent mitoses. In better differentiated tumors, distinction from benign endocervical glandular proliferations can be challenging (see discussion of EWDGAS later). Supportive immunohistochemistry includes demonstration of gastric-type differentiation by MUC6 or HIK1083 and negative p16 staining. If necessary, HPV PCR can be used in equivocal cases, which can be helpful in distinguishing GAS from other types of mucinous and/or conventional types of endocervical adenocarcinoma.

Papanicolaou smear remains the best method to screen for cervical glandular neoplasia. Cytologic features of GAS include monolayer and honeycomb sheets or 3-D clusters of columnar cells with cytologic atypia with enlarged, hyperchromatic nuclei and prominent nucleoli with occasional cells with golden-yellow cytoplasmic mucin using Papanicolaou stain.[66] Additionally, GAS may demonstrate intracytoplasmic neutrophil entrapment.[67] Screening for gastric-type mucins in cervical secretions using HIK1083-labeled latex agglutination has been attempted but has not been widely adopted.[68]

Prognosis

The prognosis of moderately and poorly differentiated GAS is generally considered poor. Compared with usual-type endocervical adenocarcinoma, gastric-type has a significantly worse 5-year disease-free survival (91% vs 42%).[69] It is estimated that only 20% to 30% of patients, regardless of stage, survive beyond 2 years.[54] At present, survival differences between EWDGAS and moderately or poorly differentiate GAS have not been demonstrated.[69]

 Differential Diagnosis

Gastric-type endocervical adenocarcinoma
- Usual-type endocervical adenocarcinoma
  - Lacks abundant mucinous cytoplasm
  - Usually strongly positive for p16 and associated with HR-HPV
  - Negative for markers of gastric differentiation
- Intestinal-type endocervical adenocarcinoma
  - Shows goblet and/or Paneth cell differentiation
  - Positive for markers of intestinal-type mucins (eg, MUC2)
  - Usually p16 positive and associated with HR-HPV
- Signet ring cell–type endocervical adenocarcinoma
  - Exclusively signet ring morphology
  - May show either intestinal or gastric-type differentiation
  - Usually p16 positive and associated with HR-HPV
- Metastatic signet ring cell carcinomas
  - Typically from breast or stomach; patient often has a history of prior malignancy
  - Lacks an identifiable in situ component
  - May be positive for GATA3 if from breast
  - Usually p16 negative

 Pathologic Key Features

- Tumors usually exhibit deeply invasive, irregularly shaped glands lined by cytologically atypical cells with frequent mitoses that elicit a desmoplastic stromal response.
- GAS demonstrates at least focal gastric-type differentiation by morphology and immunohistochemistry.
- MUC6 is often at least focally positive in GAS, whereas p16 is usually negative.

 Pitfalls

! Tumors may show only limited stromal invasion without significant desmoplastic response.

! Gastric-type differentiation may be focal.

! If p16 immunohistochemistry is equivocal, HPV PCR can be a useful confirmatory test.

EXTREMELY WELL-DIFFERENTIATED GASTRIC-TYPE ADENOCARCINOMA AND LOBULAR ENDOCERVICAL GLANDULAR HYPERPLASIA

Brief Introduction

The terms, *adenoma malignum* and *minimal deviation adenocarcinoma*, are now considered synonymous with the EWDGAS.[54] The history of the entity referred to by these terms is convoluted, especially because the gastric-type differentiation of this tumor was not appreciated until recently. Adenoma malignum was first described in 1870 by Gusserow, and the term, minimal deviation adenocarcinoma, was introduced in 1975.[70,71] The first case of adenoma malignum associated with PJS was reported in the German literature in 1969 by Kese.[11] It is estimated that fewer than 5% of women with PJS develop EWDGAS, whereas of newly diagnosed EWDGAS, approximately 10% occur in PJS patients.[18,61,72]

Early on, this entity was recognized as a highly differentiated form of endocervical adenocarcinoma with cytologic features indistinguishable from those of normal endocervical epithelium.[73] The challenging nature of the diagnosis was also appreciated, especially on cervical biopsies, because very well-differentiated tumors, initially interpreted as benign processes, were demonstrated in follow-up to have early tumor metastases with rapid spread to lymph nodes and/or generalized carcinomatosis.[73]

Based on the presence of mucinous cytoplasm, EWDGAS was initially classified as an endocervical adenocarcinoma. As is true for the less well-differentiated forms, however, the demonstration of pyloric-type mucins by histochemical or immunohistochemical stains allowed for reclassification of this entity as an adenocarcinoma showing gastric-type differentiation.

Lobular endocervical glandular hyperplasia (LEGH), alternatively known as pyloric gland metaplasia, refers to a benign glandular proliferation of the endocervix that may be seen in close proximity to GAS, has infrequently been reported to have atypical features including cytologic atypia and architectural complexity, has been shown to occasionally have mutations also identified in GASs, and rarely occurs in PJS patients with germline *STK11/LKB1* mutation in the absence of endocervical adenocarcinoma.[74–82] For these reasons, it has been hypothesized that atypical forms of LEGH may represent a precursor lesion of GAS.

Gross Features

The gross appearance of adenoma malignum is variable. In some cases, only a small granular ulceration involving endocervical mucosa may be seen (Fig. 7A). In other cases, the cervix may be partially or entirely replaced by a firm indurated mass imparting a barrel-shaped enlargement.[13] In LEGH, the cervix is typically grossly unremarkable; however, occasionally, variably sized cysts may be apparent involving up to the full thickness of the cervical wall.[83]

Microscopic Features

Microscopically, EWDGAS is defined by the presence of very well-differentiated infiltrative endocervical glands lined by columnar epithelium with copious pale or eosinophilic mucinous cytoplasm, basally oriented, mostly minimally atypical nuclei, and minimal to absent mitotic figures. Usually, however, focal high-grade cytologic atypia and mitotic activity can be identified with careful examination. Typically, the infiltrative glands show a haphazard arrangement and are found to deeply infiltrate the wall of the endocervix. The glands nearer the surface are usually irregular in shape, with some larger glands having a "lobster claw–like" outline. A desmoplastic, myxoid, or edematous stromal response, which may be focal, is usually present at the deepest extent of the invasive component. A stromal response is more notable around small, irregular clusters or single cells within stroma (see Fig. 7B–F).

On low-power examination, LEGH appears as a lobular proliferation of well demarcated endocervical glands centered on a larger duct that is in continuity with the endocervical canal (Fig. 8A). Although, occasionally, the glandular proliferation may extend deeply into the wall of the cervix, in most cases, it is limited to the inner half. The glands are generally round, but undulating contours of the gland lumens and papillary infoldings may be seen. On higher-power examination, glands are lined by a mucin-rich epithelium composed of tall columnar cells with copious pale/eosinophilic cytoplasm and bland, basally-located, round to oval nuclei. Nucleoli are generally indistinct. Rare mitoses may occur (usually <2 per 10 high-power fields) (see Fig. 8B, C). Occasionally, rupture, with a chronic inflammatory response to extravasated mucin, may be seen; this must be distinguished from a stromal desmoplastic response.[83] Conventional and atypical forms of LEGH have been described in PJS patients and in cases associated with EWDGAS.[66,77] Architectural features that warrant designation as atypical LEGH include epithelial infolding or distinct papillary projections into gland lumens, whereas atypical cytologic features include cell budding and/or exfoliation, loss of nuclear

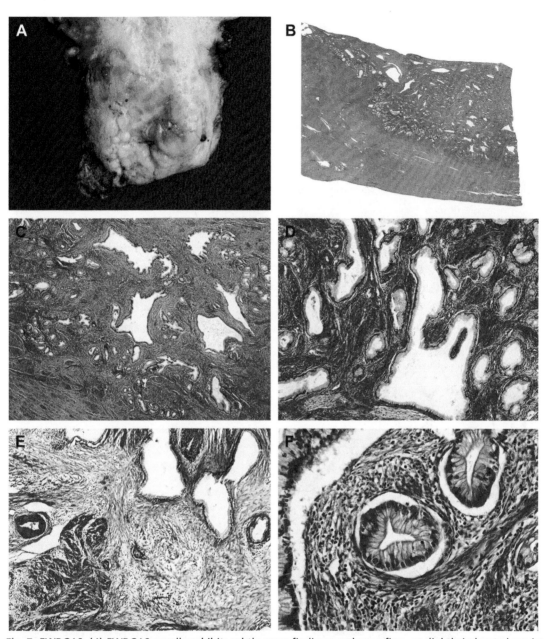

Fig. 7. EWDGAS. (*A*) EWDGAS usually exhibits subtle gross findings, such as a firm, or slightly indurated cervix; however, in some cases, only cysts and/or small areas of ulceration or erosion may be seen. (*B*) Whole-slide scan of EWDGAS that shows deep invasion of tumor into the outer third of the cervical wall. (*C*) In EWDGAS, the glandular proliferation is usually composed of both small, regular glands with bland cytology that are admixed with larger, dilated glands (H&E, 2×) with (*D*) irregular, angulated ("lobster claw-like") luminal contours (H&E, 20×). (*E*) Usually, at least focally, the pushing front of invasion shows small, angular glands and single cells with atypical cytology, usually associated with a desmoplastic stromal response that confirms the invasive and malignant nature of the proliferation (H&E, 2×). (*F*) EWDGAS shows the typical cytomorphology of proliferations with gastric-type differentiation, including abundant pale to eosinophilic cytoplasm and distinct cell borders (H&E, 40×).

polarity, nuclear enlargement and hyperchromasia, distinct nucleoli, apoptotic bodies and/or luminal debris, and apical mitoses[74,84] (see **Fig. 8D–F**).

Differential Diagnosis

EWDGAS and LEGH may show significant morphologic overlap with many of the same benign endocervical glandular proliferations. The differential

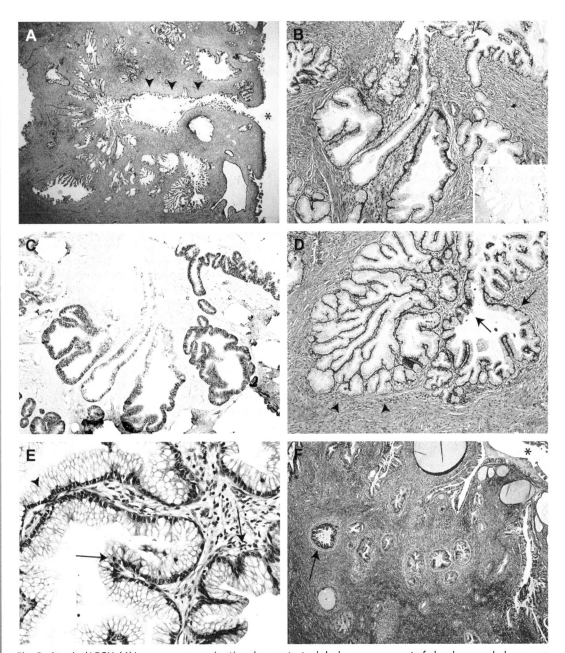

Fig. 8. Atypical LEGH. (*A*) Low-power examination demonstrates lobular arrangement of glands around a large, central duct (*arrowheads*) that is in communication with the endocervical canal (*asterisk*) (H&E, 2×). (*B*) Atypical LEGH shows features of gastric differentiation, including copious pale to eosinophilic cytoplasm (H&E, 20×) and is negative for p16 (*inset*) (p16, 20×) and (*C*) positive for MUC6 (MUC6, 20×). (*D*) Atypical LEGH (*arrows*) shows increased nuclear hyperchromasia and papillary architecture compared with adjacent nonatypical LEGH (*arrowheads*) (H&E, 20×). (*E*) Cytologically, atypical LEGH shows slight nuclear enlargement and hyperchromasia often with nucleoli (*arrow*) compared with adjacent nonatypical LEGH (*arrowhead*) (H&E, 40×). (*F*) Careful examination is always mandatory in these cases, because invasive adenocarcinoma with desmoplastic stromal response (*arrow*) can be associated with atypical forms of LEGH, which maintain a lobular arrangement about a larger duct (*asterisk*) (H&E, 2×).

diagnosis of EWDGAS includes pyloric gland metaplasia, LEGH as well as diffuse laminar endocervical glandular hyperplasia (DLEGH), endocervical adenomyoma, endocervicosis/endosalpingiosis, florid deep glands, tunnel clusters, clear cell carcinoma, and microglandular hyperplasia (Fig. 9). Pyloric gland metaplasia generally maintains the normal glandular architecture of the endocervix and is lined by epithelium that shows cytologic features of gastric-type differentiation. LEGH must be distinguished from EWDGAS, because both may appear as a proliferation of endocervical glands within endocervical stroma as well as demonstrate a remarkable lack of cytologic atypia and mitotic activity. Features that, if present, can help distinguish LEGH include (1) a lobulated glandular proliferation centered on a larger duct that is in continuity with the endocervical canal, (2) glands limited to inner one-third of endocervical stroma, (3) lack of haphazard gland arrangement, (4) no cytologic atypia, (5) no desmoplastic stromal response, (6) lack of glands in close proximity to peripheral nerves, and (7) no lymphovascular invasion.[83] DLEGH appears in the differential diagnosis with EWDGAS/LEGH because it represents a cytologically bland mucinous glandular proliferation within endocervical stroma. From low power, however, differences can be appreciated because DLEGH is usually present as a uniform laminar proliferation whereas the infiltrative glands in well-differentiated GAS are haphazard in arrangement and often extend deeply into the wall. In contrast to LEGH in which the proliferation is centered on a large duct, glands in DLEGH are present only to a uniform stromal depth and are usually limited to the inner third of the cervical wall. Additionally, DLEGH lacks evidence of gastric differentiation by immunohistochemistry.[85] Endocervical adenomyoma may be considered in the differential diagnosis of EWDGAS/LEGH based on presentation as a mass lesion and because the appearance of the benign glandular proliferation in myomatous stroma may mimic an infiltrative malignancy. Endocervical adenomyoma can be distinguished from well-differentiated GAS because the former is usually a well-circumscribed mass that shows no desmoplastic stromal reaction, and GAS lacks a smooth muscle myomatous stroma.[86] Endocervicosis and endosalpingiosis are entities to consider in the differential diagnosis of EWDGAS because these glandular proliferations may involve the outer half of the cervical wall. This location makes them suspicious for a deeply invasive malignancy; however, endocervicosis/endosalpingiosis is limited to the outer cervical wall, whereas well-differentiated GAS shows continuous infiltrative glands extending the full-thickness of the cervical wall. Endocervicosis can be further distinguished because the glandular component is unassociated with a desmoplastic stromal response despite appearing deeply situated in the endocervical stroma. Endosalpingiosis can be further distinguished because the epithelium lacks mucin and demonstrates ciliated and secretory cells typical of tubal epithelium.[87] Florid deep glands are a benign proliferation of typically rounded glands lined by endocervical-type epithelium that may involve deep endocervical stroma and thus may mimic EWDGAS. The epithelium in florid deep glands may show variable amounts of pale mucinous cytoplasm with minimal cytologic atypia and absent mitoses, causing further confusion with EWDGAS.[88] However, EWDGAS shows at least focal cytologic atypia and/or a desmoplastic stromal response and is positive for markers of gastric differentiation. The lobular architecture, bland cytomorphology, and occasional evidence of gastric differentiation of tunnel clusters may mimic EWDGAS/LEGH. Tunnel clusters can usually be distinguished, however, due to (1) relative focal distribution and circumscribed nature, (2) superficial location in cervical stroma, and (3) epithelium lining the cystic glands that is variable in appearance with a typical columnar mucinous lining (type A tunnel clusters) and an attenuated mucinous epithelium (type B tunnel clusters). LEGH appears less circumscribed as a proliferation centered on a larger duct and lacks the attenuated epithelial component. The gland contours of EWDGAS are typically more irregular than seen in tunnel clusters and generally also lack the attenuated epithelial component. Rarely, type A tunnel clusters may show cytologic atypia; however, this atypia is not associated with appreciable mitotic activity. With thorough examination, at least focal cytologic atypia can usually be found in EWDGAS that is associated with mitotic activity.[89,90] Clear cell adenocarcinoma usually is easily distinguished from EWDGAS/LEGH based on its typical combination of architectural patterns, including tubulocystic, papillary, and solid areas, often with a desmoplastic stromal response as well as overtly malignant cytologic features.

Diagnosis

A diagnosis of EWDGAS is based entirely on the morphologic findings of extremely well-differentiated epithelial glands haphazardly invading endocervical stroma. When present, deep stromal invasion can be helpful in distinguishing EWDGAS from benign mimics. The confirmation of gastric differentiation can be helpful but does not exclude the possibility of LEGH. By immunohistochemistry, p16 is generally negative, and HR-HPV is not detected.

LEGH also shows evidence of gastric differentiation; however, a helpful diagnostic feature is the low-power observation of the glandular proliferation centered on a large duct. Atypical architectural and cytologic features may be seen in LEGH and are considered features of a precursor lesion.

Prognosis

Like the moderately and poorly differentiated GASs, the prognosis of EWDGAS is generally

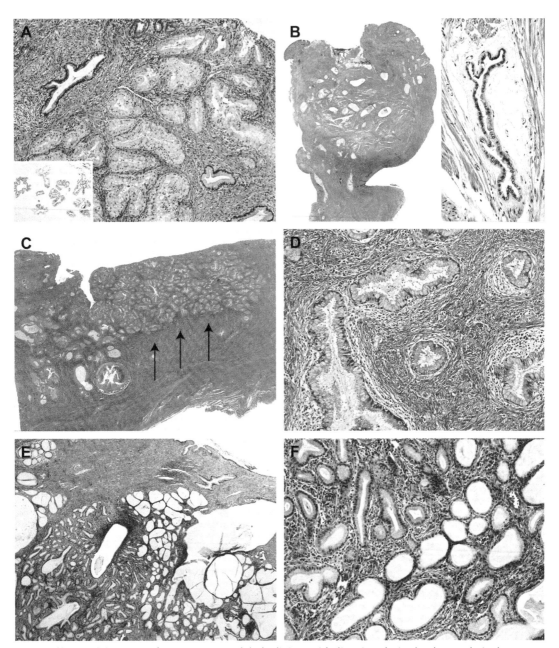

Fig. 9. Differential diagnosis of LEGH/EWDGAS. (*A*) The lining epithelium in pyloric gland metaplasia shows cytologic features of gastric-type differentiation (H&E, 10×) and positivity for MUC6 (*inset*) (MUC6, 10×). (*B*, left image, whole slide scan) The macroscopic appearance of endocervical adenomyoma is typically an exophytic, mass lesion, in contrast to LEGH/EWDGAS; however, (right image, H&E, 40×) the bland endocervical epithelial component in myomatous stroma may closely mimic and invasive process. (*C*) Low-power examination of an endocervical glandular proliferation showing uniform depth of extension (*arrow*) is in keeping with DLEGH (H&E, whole slide scan). (*D*) Higher-power examination of DLEGH shows more conventional endocervical epithelium without gastric-type differentiation that is negative for MUC6 (H&E, 20×). (*E*) Tunnel clusters classically appear as a lobular proliferation of endocervical-type glands in superficial endocervical stroma and rarely show deep involvement of the cervical wall (H&E, 2×). (*F*) Tunnel clusters can be distinguished based on the presence of characteristic mixture of noncystic glands (type A tunnel clusters) and cystically dilated glands with attenuated epithelium (type B tunnel clusters) (H&E, 10×).

considered poor.[54] Most patients experience recurrence of tumor within 2 years of diagnosis.[61] Compared with conventional-type endocervical adenocarcinoma, GAS has a worse 5-year disease-free survival (74% vs 30%).[54]

Historically, it was thought that endocervical adenocarcinoma occurring in a PJS patient behaved more aggressively. Studies in sporadic EWDGAS have preliminarily shown, however, that the worse prognosis is more likely attributable to mutation in *STK11/LKB1*.[24]

RECOMMENDATIONS FOR SCREENING, MANAGEMENT, AND ADDITIONAL GENETIC TESTING

In the context of the topics discussed, there are 2 situations in which practicing surgical pathologists may choose to make management recommendations or suggest additional genetic testing. The first situation occurs when a pathologist encounters a gynecologic neoplasm in a specimen from

---

Pathologic Key Features

- LEGH is a lobular proliferation centered on a large duct that is in continuity with the endocervical canal; if it shows atypical features, it is likely a precursor lesion of GAS.

- Atypical architectural features in LEGH include epithelial infolding or distinct papillary projections into gland lumens. Atypical cytologic features in LEGH include cell budding and/or exfoliation, loss of nuclear polarity, nuclear enlargement and hyperchromasia, distinct nucleoli, apoptotic bodies and/or luminal debris, and apical mitoses.

- Complete surgical excision is warranted for atypical features in LEGH.

- Deeply invasive haphazard glands that, at least focally, exhibit malignant cytologic features and a desmoplastic stromal response are the most helpful features in diagnosing EWDGAS. Lymphovascular invasion can help confirm malignancy.

Differential Diagnosis

Lobular endocervical glandular hyperplasia
- Glandular proliferation centered on a larger duct that is in continuity with the endocervical canal

- Glands limited to inner wall of the endocervix

- Lack of haphazard arrangement of glands

- No cytologic atypia

- No desmoplastic stromal response

- No lymphovascular invasion

Diffuse laminar endocervical glandular hyperplasia

- Bandlike arrangement of endocervical-type glands in relatively superficial endocervical stroma (inner one-third of wall) that shows a uniform and sharply demarcated deepest extent of proliferating glands

- Negative for markers of gastric differentiation (eg, HIK1083)

Endocervical adenomyoma

- Usually a well-circumscribed mass

- Lacks desmoplastic stromal reaction and has characteristic myomatous stroma

Endocervicosis

- Glandular proliferation of endocervical-type centered in the outer half of the cervical wall
- No associated desmoplastic stromal response
- Benign cytologic features

Endosalpingiosis

- Glandular proliferation centered in the outer half of the cervical wall
- No associated desmoplastic stromal response
- Banal lining epithelium has secretory and ciliated cells typical of tubal epithelium

Florid deep glands

- Typically rounded glands present in deep endocervical stroma
- Variable amounts of pale mucinous cytoplasm with minimal cytologic atypia and rare to absent mitoses
- No desmoplastic stromal response
- No evidence of gastric differentiation

Tunnel clusters

- Usually relatively focal and circumscribed proliferation
- Lined by columnar or attenuated banal appearing epithelium

Clear cell adenocarcinoma

- Usually demonstrates combination of architectural patterns, including tubulocystic, papillary, and solid
- Usually associated with a desmoplastic stromal response
- Malignant cytologic features

Pitfalls

! Cytologic atypia in EWDGAS may be focal.

! Before making a diagnosis of EWDGAS, always consider the diagnostic possibility of endocervical adenomyoma.

a woman with an established diagnosis of PJS. PJS-associated ovarian neoplasia is usually managed similarly to sporadic forms. SCTAT is often managed akin to similar stage granulosa cell tumors; however, because SCTAT associated with PJS demonstrates a nearly universally benign clinical course, some investigators have suggested less aggressive management. GAS associated with PJS is also managed similarly to the sporadic form. In the setting of a diagnosis of atypical LEGH, the authors suggest including a

recommendation for complete surgical excision based on accumulating data supporting the hypothesis that atypical LEGH represents a precursor of GAS.

The second situation occurs when a pathologist renders a diagnosis, such as those discussed previously, in a patient who does not have an established diagnosis of PJS. In this case, due to the variable and broad clinical presentation of PJS, the authors suggest noting the association between the diagnosed neoplasm and PJS and recommending appropriate additional testing of the patient and possibly family members as clinically indicated.

There are no established guidelines for screening for gynecologic neoplasia in PJS patients. PJS patients should continue with routine cervical cytology screening, and, ideally, the diagnosis of PJS is provided to the reviewing cytotechnologist/cytopathologist so that careful review for features of GAS can be performed. Beyond routine cervical cytology screening, some investigators advocate for yearly pelvic examinations and/or ultrasound beginning in young adulthood to detect ovarian neoplasia; however, this recommendation has not been uniformly accepted.[2,3]

REFERENCES

1. Jeghers H, McKusick KV, Katz KH. Generalized intestinal polyposis and melanin spots of the oral mucosa, lips and digits; a syndrome of diagnostic significance. N Engl J Med 1949;241(26):1031–6.
2. Riegert-Johnson D, Ferga CG, Westra W, et al. Peutz-jeghers syndrome. In: Riegert-Johnson DL, Boardman LA, Hefferon T, et al, editors. Cancer syndromes. Bethesda (MD): National Center for Biotechnology Information; 2009.
3. McGarrity TJ, Kulin HE, Zaino RJ. Peutz-Jeghers syndrome. Am J Gastroenterol 2000;95(3):596–604.
4. Weber RA. The coincidence of perioral pigmented spots and small bowel polyps. Ann Surg 1954; 140(6):901–5.
5. Bartholomew LG, Dahlin DC, Waugh JM. Intestinal polyposis associated with mucocutaneous melanin pigmentation (Peutz-Jeghers syndrome). Proc Staff Meet Mayo Clin 1957;32(24):675–80.
6. Dormandy TL. Gastrointestinal polyposis with mucocutaneous pigmentation (Peutz-Jeghers syndrome). N Engl J Med 1957;256(25):1186–90.
7. #175200 Peutz-Jeghers Syndrome. PJS. 2015. Available at: http://www.omim.org/entry/175200. Accessed September 1, 2015.
8. Scully RE. Sex cord tumor with annular tubules a distinctive ovarian tumor of the Peutz-Jeghers syndrome. Cancer 1970;25(5):1107–21.
9. Zung A, Shoham Z, Open M, et al. Sertoli cell tumor causing precocious puberty in a girl with Peutz-Jeghers syndrome. Gynecol Oncol 1998;70(3): 421–4.
10. Cantu JM, Rivera H, Ocampo-Campos R, et al. Peutz-Jeghers syndrome with feminizing sertoli cell tumor. Cancer 1980;46(1):223–8.
11. Kese G. Adenocarcinoma of the cervix uteri in a 28-year-old woman with Peutz-Jeghers syndrome. Zentralbl Gynakol 1969;91(7):215–8, [in German].
12. McGowan L, Young RH, Scully RE. Peutz-Jeghers syndrome with "adenoma malignum" of the cervix. A report of two cases. Gynecol Oncol 1980;10(2): 125–33.
13. Young RH, Welch WR, Dickersin GR, et al. Ovarian sex cord tumor with annular tubules: review of 74 cases including 27 with Peutz-Jeghers syndrome and four with adenoma malignum of the cervix. Cancer 1982;50(7):1384–402.
14. Beggs AD, Latchford AR, Vasen HF, et al. Peutz-Jeghers syndrome: a systematic review and recommendations for management. Gut 2010;59(7):975–86.
15. Hemminki A. The molecular basis and clinical aspects of Peutz-Jeghers syndrome. Cell Mol Life Sci 1999;55(5):735–50.
16. Hemminki A, Tomlinson I, Markie D, et al. Localization of a susceptibility locus for Peutz-Jeghers syndrome to 19p using comparative genomic hybridization and targeted linkage analysis. Nat Genet 1997;15(1): 87–90.
17. Jenne DE, Reimann H, Nezu J, et al. Peutz-Jeghers syndrome is caused by mutations in a novel serine threonine kinase. Nat Genet 1998;18(1):38–43.
18. Banno K, Kisu I, Yanokura M, et al. Hereditary gynecological tumors associated with Peutz-Jeghers syndrome (Review). Oncol Lett 2013;6(5):1184–8.
19. Hernan I, Roig I, Martin B, et al. De novo germline mutation in the serine-threonine kinase STK11/LKB1 gene associated with Peutz-Jeghers syndrome. Clin Genet 2004;66(1):58–62.
20. Ollila S, Makela TP. The tumor suppressor kinase LKB1: lessons from mouse models. J Mol Cell Biol 2011;3(6):330–40.
21. Katajisto P, Vallenius T, Vaahtomeri K, et al. The LKB1 tumor suppressor kinase in human disease. Biochim Biophys Acta 2007;1775(1):63–75.
22. Hardie DG. Minireview: the AMP-activated protein kinase cascade: the key sensor of cellular energy status. Endocrinology 2003;144(12):5179–83.
23. Vaahtomeri K, Makela TP. Molecular mechanisms of tumor suppression by LKB1. FEBS Lett 2011;585(7): 944–51.
24. Kuragaki C, Enomoto T, Ueno Y, et al. Mutations in the STK11 gene characterize minimal deviation adenocarcinoma of the uterine cervix. Lab Invest 2003;83(1):35–45.
25. Avizienyte E, Roth S, Loukola A, et al. Somatic mutations in LKB1 are rare in sporadic colorectal and testicular tumors. Cancer Res 1998;58(10): 2087–90.
26. Bignell GR, Barfoot R, Seal S, et al. Low frequency of somatic mutations in the LKB1/Peutz-Jeghers syndrome gene in sporadic breast cancer. Cancer Res 1998;58(7):1384–6.
27. Resta N, Simone C, Mareni C, et al. STK11 mutations in Peutz-Jeghers syndrome and sporadic colon cancer. Cancer Res 1998;58(21):4799–801.
28. Ji H, Ramsey MR, Hayes DN, et al. LKB1 modulates lung cancer differentiation and metastasis. Nature 2007;448(7155):807–10.
29. Wingo SN, Gallardo TD, Akbay EA, et al. Somatic LKB1 mutations promote cervical cancer progression. PLoS One 2009;4(4):e5137.
30. Kato N, Romero M, Catasus L, et al. The STK11/LKB1 Peutz-Jegher gene is not involved in the pathogenesis of sporadic sex cord-stromal tumors, although loss of heterozygosity at 19p13.3 indicates other gene alteration in these tumors. Hum Pathol 2004;35(9):1101–4.
31. Mehenni H, Blouin JL, Radhakrishna U, et al. Peutz-Jeghers syndrome: confirmation of linkage to chromosome 19p13.3 and identification of a potential

second locus, on 19q13.4. Am J Hum Genet 1997;
61(6):1327–34.

32. Buchet-Poyau K, Mehenni H, Radhakrishna U, et al. Search for the second Peutz-Jeghers syndrome locus: exclusion of the STK13, PRKCG, KLK10, and PSCD2 genes on chromosome 19 and the STK11IP gene on chromosome 2. Cytogenet Genome Res 2002;97(3–4):171–8.

33. Hearle N, Lucassen A, Wang R, et al. Mapping of a translocation breakpoint in a Peutz-Jeghers hamartoma to the putative PJS locus at 19q13.4 and mutation analysis of candidate genes in polyp and STK11-negative PJS cases. Genes Chromosomes Cancer 2004;41(2):163–9.

34. Alhopuro P, Katajisto P, Lehtonen R, et al. Mutation analysis of three genes encoding novel LKB1-interacting proteins, BRG1, STRADalpha, and MO25alpha, in Peutz-Jeghers syndrome. Br J Cancer 2005;92(6):1126–9.

35. de Leng WW, Keller JJ, Luiten S, et al. STRAD in Peutz-Jeghers syndrome and sporadic cancers. J Clin Pathol 2005;58(10):1091–5.

36. Young RH. Sex cord-stromal tumors of the ovary and testis: their similarities and differences with consideration of selected problems. Mod Pathol 2005; 18(Suppl 2):S81–98.

37. Lele SM, Sawh RN, Zaharopoulos P, et al. Malignant ovarian sex cord tumor with annular tubules in a patient with Peutz-Jeghers syndrome: a case report. Mod Pathol 2000;13(4):466–70.

38. Barker D, Sharma R, McIndoe A, et al. An unusual case of sex cord tumor with annular tubules with malignant transformation in a patient with Peutz-Jeghers syndrome. Int J Gynecol Pathol 2010; 29(1):27–32.

39. Rodu B, Martinez MG Jr. Peutz-Jeghers syndrome and cancer. Oral Surg Oral Med Oral Pathol 1984; 58(5):584–8.

40. Connolly DC, Katabuchi H, Cliby WA, et al. Somatic mutations in the STK11/LKB1 gene are uncommon in rare gynecological tumor types associated with Peutz-Jegher's syndrome. Am J Pathol 2000; 156(1):339–45.

41. Tavassoli FA, Norris HJ. Sertoli tumors of the ovary. A clinicopathologic study of 28 cases with ultrastructural observations. Cancer 1980;46(10):2281–97.

42. Hart WR, Kumar N, Crissman JD. Ovarian neoplasms resembling sex cord tumors with annular tubules. Cancer 1980;45(9):2352–63.

43. Czernobilsky B, Gaedcke G, Dallenbach-Hellweg G. Endometrioid differentiation in ovarian sex cord tumor with annular tubules accompanied by gestagenic effect. Cancer 1985;55(4):738–44.

44. Scully RE. Gonadoblastoma. A review of 74 cases. Cancer 1970;25(6):1340–56.

45. Geiersbach KB, Jarboe EA, Jahromi MS, et al. FOXL2 mutation and large-scale genomic imbalances in adult granulosa cell tumors of the ovary. Cancer Genet 2011;204(11):596–602.

46. Guerrieri C, Frånlund B, Malmström H, et al. Ovarian endometrioid carcinomas simulating sex cord-stromal tumors: a study using inhibin and cytokeratin 7. Int J Gynecol Pathol 1998;17(3):266–71.

47. Movahedi-Lankarani S, Kurman RJ. Calretinin, a more sensitive but less specific marker than alpha-inhibin for ovarian sex cord-stromal neoplasms: an immunohistochemical study of 215 cases. Am J Surg Pathol 2002;26(11):1477–83.

48. Deavers MT, Malpica A, Ordonez NG, et al. Ovarian steroid cell tumors: an immunohistochemical study including a comparison of calretinin with inhibin. Int J Gynecol Pathol 2003;22(2):162–7.

49. Yazdi HM. Fine needle aspiration cytology of ovarian sex cord tumor with annular tubules. Acta Cytol 1987;31(3):340–4.

50. Gloor E. Ovarian sex cord tumor with annular tubules. Clinicopathologic report of two benign and one malignant cases with long follow-ups. Virchows Arch A Pathol Anat Histol 1979;384(2):185–93.

51. Ahn GH, Chi JG, Lee SK. Ovarian sex cord tumor with annular tubules. Cancer 1986;57(5):1066–73.

52. Shen K, Wu PC, Lang JH, et al. Ovarian sex cord tumor with annular tubules: a report of six cases. Gynecol Oncol 1993;48(2):180–4.

53. Young RH, Scully RE. Ovarian Sertoli cell tumors: a report of 10 cases. Int J Gynecol Pathol 1984;2(4): 349–63.

54. Kurman RJ, Carcangiu ML, Herrington CS, et al. WHO classification of tumours of female reproductive organs. In: Bosman FT, Jaffe ES, Lakhani SR, et al, editors. WHO classification of tumours. 4th edition. Lyon (France): International Agency for Research on Cancer; 2014. p. 183–94.

55. Oliva E, Alvarez T, Young RH. Sertoli cell tumors of the ovary: a clinicopathologic and immunohistochemical study of 54 cases. Am J Surg Pathol 2005;29(2):143–56.

56. Korzets A, Nouriel H, Steiner Z, et al. Resistant hypertension associated with a renin-producing ovarian Sertoli cell tumor. Am J Clin Pathol 1986;85(2):242–7.

57. Ishihara K, Kurihara M, Goso Y, et al. Peripheral alpha-linked N-acetylglucosamine on the carbohydrate moiety of mucin derived from mammalian gastric gland mucous cells: epitope recognized by a newly characterized monoclonal antibody. Biochem J 1996;318(Pt 2):409–16.

58. Ishii K, Hosaka N, Toki T, et al. A new view of the so-called adenoma malignum of the uterine cervix. Virchows Arch 1998;432(4):315–22.

59. Kusanagi Y, Kojima A, Mikami Y, et al. Absence of high-risk human papillomavirus (HPV) detection in endocervical adenocarcinoma with gastric morphology and phenotype. Am J Pathol 2010; 177(5):2169–75.

60. Xu JY, Hashi A, Kondo T, et al. Absence of human papillomavirus infection in minimal deviation adenocarcinoma and lobular endocervical glandular hyperplasia. Int J Gynecol Pathol 2005;24(3): 296–302.

61. Gilks CB, Young RH, Aguirre P, et al. Adenoma malignum (minimal deviation adenocarcinoma) of the uterine cervix. A clinicopathological and immunohistochemical analysis of 26 cases. Am J Surg Pathol 1989;13(9):717–29.

62. Kojima A, Mikami Y, Sudo T, et al. Gastric morphology and immunophenotype predict poor outcome in mucinous adenocarcinoma of the uterine cervix. Am J Surg Pathol 2007;31(5):664–72.

63. Mikami Y, McCluggage WG. Endocervical glandular lesions exhibiting gastric differentiation: an emerging spectrum of benign, premalignant, and malignant lesions. Adv Anat Pathol 2013;20(4): 227–37.

64. McCluggage WG, Shah R, Connolly LE, et al. Intestinal-type cervical adenocarcinoma in situ and adenocarcinoma exhibit a partial enteric immunophenotype with consistent expression of CDX2. Int J Gynecol Pathol 2008;27(1):92–100.

65. Saad RS, Ghorab Z, Khalifa MA, et al. CDX2 as a marker for intestinal differentiation: Its utility and limitations. World J Gastrointest Surg 2011;3(11): 159–66.

66. Kondo T, Hashi A, Murata S, et al. Endocervical adenocarcinomas associated with lobular endocervical glandular hyperplasia: a report of four cases with histochemical and immunohistochemical analyses. Mod Pathol 2005;18(9):1199–210.

67. Kawakami F, Mikami Y, Sudo T, et al. Cytologic features of gastric-type adenocarcinoma of the uterine cervix. Diagn Cytopathol 2015;43(10):791–6.

68. Omori M, Hashi A, Ishii Y, et al. Clinical impact of preoperative screening for gastric mucin secretion in cervical discharge by HIK1083-labeled latex agglutination test. Am J Clin Pathol 2008;130(4): 585–94.

69. Karamurzin YS, Kiyokawa T, Parkash V, et al. Gastric-type endocervical adenocarcinoma: an aggressive tumor with unusual metastatic patterns and poor prognosis. Am J Surg Pathol 2015; 39(11):1449–57.

70. Silverberg SG, Hurt WG. Minimal deviation adenocarcinoma ("adenoma malignum") of the cervix: a reappraisal. Am J Obstet Gynecol 1975;121(7):971–5.

71. Srivatsa PJ, Keeney GL, Podratz KC. Disseminated cervical adenoma malignum and bilateral ovarian sex cord tumors with annular tubules associated with Peutz-Jeghers syndrome. Gynecol Oncol 1994;53(2):256–64.

72. Spigelman AD, Murday V, Phillips RK. Cancer and the Peutz-Jeghers syndrome. Gut 1989;30(11): 1588–90.

73. McKelvey J, Goodlin R. Adenoma malignum of the cervix A cancer of deceptively innocent histologic findings. Cancer 1963;16:549–57.

74. Mikami Y, Kiyokawa T, Hata S, et al. Gastrointestinal immunophenotype in adenocarcinomas of the uterine cervix and related glandular lesions: a possible link between lobular endocervical glandular hyperplasia/pyloric gland metaplasia and 'adenoma malignum'. Mod Pathol 2004;17(8):962–72.

75. Matsubara A, Sekine S, Ogawa R, et al. Lobular endocervical glandular hyperplasia is a neoplastic entity with frequent activating GNAS mutations. Am J Surg Pathol 2014;38(3):370–6.

76. Hirasawa A, Akahane T, Tsuruta T, et al. Lobular endocervical glandular hyperplasia and peritoneal pigmentation associated with Peutz-Jeghers syndrome due to a germline mutation of STK11. Ann Oncol 2012;23(11):2990–2.

77. Sugihara T, Nakagawa S, Sasajima Y, et al. Case of minimal deviation adenocarcinoma: possible clinical link to lobular endocervical glandular hyperplasia as its origin. J Obstet Gynaecol Res 2015;41(3): 483–7.

78. Takei Y, Fujiwara H, Nagashima T, et al. Successful pregnancy in a Peutz-Jeghers syndrome patient with lobular endocervical glandular hyperplasia. J Obstet Gynaecol Res 2015;41(3):468–73.

79. Kawauchi S, Kusuda T, Liu XP, et al. Is lobular endocervical glandular hyperplasia a cancerous precursor of minimal deviation adenocarcinoma?: a comparative molecular-genetic and immunohistochemical study. Am J Surg Pathol 2008;32(12): 1807–15.

80. Nishio S, Tsuda H, Fujiyoshi N, et al. Clinicopathological significance of cervical adenocarcinoma associated with lobular endocervical glandular hyperplasia. Pathol Res Pract 2009;205(5):331–7.

81. Nara M, Hashi A, Murata S, et al. Lobular endocervical glandular hyperplasia as a presumed precursor of cervical adenocarcinoma independent of human papillomavirus infection. Gynecol Oncol 2007; 106(2):289–98.

82. Tsuji T, Togami S, Nomoto M, et al. Uterine cervical carcinomas associated with lobular endocervical glandular hyperplasia. Histopathology 2011;59(1): 55–62.

83. Nucci MR, Clement PB, Young RH. Lobular endocervical glandular hyperplasia, not otherwise specified: a clinicopathologic analysis of thirteen cases of a distinctive pseudoneoplastic lesion and comparison with fourteen cases of adenoma malignum. Am J Surg Pathol 1999;23(8):886–91.

84. Ito M, Minamiguchi S, Mikami Y, et al. Peutz-Jeghers syndrome-associated atypical mucinous proliferation of the uterine cervix: a case of minimal deviation adenocarcinoma ('adenoma malignum') in situ. Pathol Res Pract 2012;208(10):623–7.

85. Jones MA, Young RH, Scully RE. Diffuse laminar endocervical glandular hyperplasia. A benign lesion often confused with adenoma malignum (minimal deviation adenocarcinoma). Am J Surg Pathol 1991;15(12):1123–9.

86. Gilks CB, Young RH, Clement PB, et al. Adenomyomas of the uterine cervix of of endocervical type: a report of ten cases of a benign cervical tumor that may be confused with adenoma malignum [corrected]. Mod Pathol 1996;9(3):220–4.

87. Young RH, Clement PB. Endocervicosis involving the uterine cervix: a report of four cases of a benign process that may be confused with deeply invasive endocervical adenocarcinoma. Int J Gynecol Pathol 2000;19(4):322–8.

88. Daya D, Young RH. Florid deep glands of the uterine cervix. Another mimic of adenoma malignum. Am J Clin Pathol 1995;103(5):614–7.

89. Jones MA, Young RH. Endocervical type A (noncystic) tunnel clusters with cytologic atypia. A report of 14 cases. Am J Surg Pathol 1996;20(11):1312–8.

90. Young RH, Clement PB. Pseudoneoplastic glandular lesions of the uterine cervix. Semin Diagn Pathol 1991;8(4):234–49.

Gynecologic Manifestations of Less Commonly Encountered Hereditary Syndromes

Deborah F. DeLair, MD, Robert A. Soslow, MD*

KEYWORDS

- Hereditary leiomyomatosis renal cell carcinoma syndrome • Tuberous sclerosis • von Hippel-Lindau
- Nevoid basal cell carcinoma syndrome • Cowden syndrome • Ollier disease • Maffucci syndrome
- Carney complex

ABSTRACT

This review covers gynecologic manifestations that may occur in rare hereditary syndromes. Recent advances in disorders, such as hereditary leiomyomatosis, renal cell carcinoma syndrome and tuberous sclerosis complex, are discussed as well as lesions that occur in von Hippel-Lindau syndrome, nevoid basal cell carcinoma syndrome, Cowden syndrome, Ollier disease/Maffucci syndrome, and Carney complex. Characteristic clinicopathologic features of each of these syndromes are discussed with an emphasis on the key features that enable pathologists to identify patients at highest risk for these diseases.

HEREDITARY LEIOMYOMATOSIS RENAL CELL CARCINOMA SYNDROME

Hereditary leiomyomatosis renal cell carcinoma syndrome (HLRCC) is an autosomal dominant syndrome due to a germline mutation in the *fumarate hydratase* (*FH*) gene located on chromosome 1q42.3. The syndrome predisposes patients to an aggressive form of renal cancer as well as uterine and cutaneous leiomyomas that have underlying *FH* abnormalities[1–3] (Table 1). The incidence of the syndrome is not definitively known but is estimated to be 1 in 10,000 to 50,000 individuals.[4] Virtually all women with HLRCC develop uterine and cutaneous leiomyomas whereas the penetrance for renal cell carcinoma (RCC) is approximately 20% to 30%.[5] Although leiomyomas with

FH abnormalities (L-FHs) occur in almost all patients with HLRCC, they can also be sporadic and can occur in patients without the syndrome.[6]

CLINICAL FEATURES

The median age at diagnosis for L-FHs in HLRCC is approximately 30 years compared with sporadic leiomyomas, which usually present a decade later. Patients often have multiple, large, and symptomatic leiomyomas, which often lead to hysterectomy at an early age.[7–9] Occasionally, a patient may present with uterine leiomyomas as the initial manifestation of the syndrome.[2,8] Frequently, patients do not have a family history suggestive of HLRCC because the penetrance is incomplete and variable.[5]

GROSS/MICROSCOPIC FEATURES AND DIAGNOSIS

There have been a handful of studies that have examined the morphologic features that are present in L-FHs.[4,7,10,11] Grossly, L-FHs are similar to leiomyomas without FH abnormalities but are often multiple and large. Microscopically, the tumors have an eosinophilic, epithelioid, and sometimes cellular appearance at low power. The cells show a fascicular growth pattern and the background vasculature is staghorn or pericytomatous. The nuclei are ovoid to round with a vesicular appearance and optical clearing and have inclusion-like nucleoli with perinuclear halos (Fig. 1A). Usually the cells have little to no atypia; however, the atypia may be severe and diffuse,

Department of Pathology, Memorial Sloan Kettering Cancer Center, 1275 York Avenue, New York, NY 10065, USA
* Corresponding author.
E-mail address: soslowr@mskcc.org

Surgical Pathology 9 (2016) 269–287
http://dx.doi.org/10.1016/j.path.2016.01.008
1875-9181/16/$ – see front matter © 2016 Elsevier Inc. All rights reserved.

Table 1
Diagnostic criteria for proposed for hereditary leiomyomatosis renal cell carcinoma syndrome as proposed by Smit and colleagues[3]

Major Criteria	Minor Criteria
Multiple cutaneous leiomyomas	Surgical resection of severely symptomatic uterine leiomyomas before age 40
	Type 2 papillary or collecting duct RCC before age 40
	First-degree family member with any major or minor criteria

The diagnosis requires 1 major criteria or 2 minor criteria.

From Smit DL, Mensenkamp AR, Badeloe S, et al. Hereditary leiomyomatosis and renal cell cancer in families referred for fumarate hydratase germline mutation analysis. Clin Genet 2011;79(1):49–59.

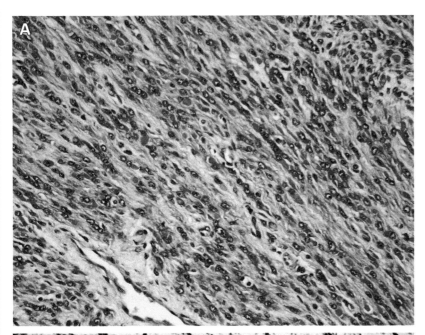

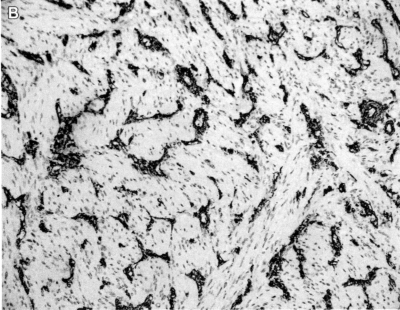

Fig. 1. (*A*) Uterine leiomyoma with FH abnormality. Morphologic features include an epithelioid appearance, prominent nucleoli with perinucleolar halos, and fibrillary cytoplasm with pink globules. (*B*) Leiomyoma with immunohistochemistry for fumarate hydratase. Loss of staining indicates an *FH* abnormality. Note the internal control in the form of vessels. (*Courtesy of* Dr Karuna Garg, University of California, San Francisco.)

similar to that seen in atypical or bizarre leiomyomas. The cytoplasm has a fibrillary appearance, which aggregates to form pink globules.

Immunohistochemistry also may be used to identify L-FHs. When there is a defect in the *FH* gene, fumarate accumulates, which in turn reacts with cysteine to form 2-succinocysteine (2SC). Increased levels of 2SC in the cell can then be detected by immunohistochemistry. This antibody has been shown to be a sensitive and specific biomarker in L-FHs and correlates well with morphology.[4,11,12] Unfortunately, this antibody is currently not commercially available. The antibody for FH also has been used as a biomarker and expression is usually lost (see **Fig.** 1B) but this has been shown less sensitive than 2SC. The morphologic and immunophenotypic features of L-FHs do not differentiate, however, between somatic and germline origin.

DIFFERENTIAL DIAGNOSIS

The differential diagnosis of a leiomyoma with FH abnormalities includes other tumors with smooth muscle differentiation, including leiomyoma (**Box 1**), leiomyosarcoma, and perivascular epithelioid cell tumor (PEComa).[4] Morphologic features useful in differentiating an epithelioid leiomyoma from L-FHs include staghorn/pericytomatous vasculature, eosinophilic globules, and prominent nucleoli with perinucleolar halos, which are absent in the former. In addition, epithelioid leiomyomas show true epithelioid cells whereas in L-FHs, the cells are pseudoepithelioid, with round to ovid nuclei but with a spindle-shaped cytoplasm. Leiomyosarcoma should be considered if atypia is severe and diffuse but L-FHs do not show the coagulative necrosis and mitotic activity required for that diagnosis. Finally, PEComa shows smooth muscle differentiation, staghorn/pericytomatous vasculature, and an epithelioid appearance, but specific morphologic features seen in PEComa (discussed later) as well as immunoreactivity for human melanoma black 45 (HMB-45) and melan-A help distinguish the 2 entities.

PROGNOSIS

Leiomyomas that occur in the setting of HLRCC are benign; however, leiomyosarcomas have also been reported in patients with the syndrome.[13] Prognosis of patients with HLRCC is largely dependent on the RCCs that occur in HLRCC because they are clinically aggressive, often present at advanced stage, and cause significant morbidity and mortality.[5] Because leiomyomas in patients with HLRCC occur approximately a decade before the age of onset of RCC, the recognition of the morphologic features may aid in identifying these patients before they develop RCC.

TUBEROUS SCLEROSIS COMPLEX

Tuberous sclerosis complex (TSC) is an autosomal dominant syndrome characterized by a germline mutation in *TSC1* or *TSC2* on chromosomes 9q34 and 16p13, respectively. The estimated prevalence of TSC is approximately 1 in 6000 to 9000 people and mutations in the *TSC2* gene account for up to 90% of cases.[14] TSC is a neurocutaneous, multisystem disease with cellular hyperplasia and tissue dysplasia with variable clinical phenotypes. Some of the major diagnostic criteria include cardiac rhabdomyomas, cutaneous and mucosal hypopigmented macules and angiofibromas, cortical dysplasia (tubers), subependymal giant cell astrocytoma, and retinal

---

Box 1
Key features of leiomyomas associated with hereditary leiomyomatosis renal cell carcinoma

	Hereditary Leiomyomatosis Renal Cell Carcinoma Leiomyomas	Non–Fumarate Hydratase–Deficient Sporadic Leiomyomas
Mean age at diagnosis	30	40
No. of leiomyomas	Always multiple	Single and multiple
Symptomatic	Yes	Variable
Cell shape	Epithelioid/spindled	Typically spindled
Vasculature	Frequently staghorn/ pericytomatous	Thick-walled
Prominent nucleoli/ perinucleolar halos	Yes	No
Cytoplasmic globules	Yes	No
Immunohistochemistry	FH lost, 2-Succinocysteine +	FH retained, 2-Succinocysteine −

hamartomas (Table 2). One of the other diagnostic hallmarks of TSC includes a family of mesenchymal tumors with perivascular epithelioid cell (PEC) differentiation, including angiomyolipoma, lymphangioleiomyomatosis (LAM), and PEComa. All 3 of these entities have been described as occurring in the female genital tract in women with and without TSC.[15–26]

LYMPHANGIOLEIOMYOMATOSIS

LAM is a hamartomatous proliferation of cells with myomelanocytic differentiation around lymphatic vessels that causes dilatation of lymphatic spaces. In the lung, it progressively destroys lung parenchyma and may lead to respiratory insufficiency and death. LAM also frequently occurs in mediastinal, retroperitoneal, and axial lymph nodes as well as gynecologic organs, usually the uterus.

Microscopically, LAM cells show spindled to epithelioid-shaped cells with round to ovoid nuclei and pale to eosinophilic cytoplasm. The cells are arranged in fascicles and form nodules with abundant cleftlike spaces that may be irregularly dilated (Fig. 2A). In a study comparing sporadic LAM to LAM associated with TSC, Hayashi and colleagues[18] found morphologic and topographic differences in sporadic LAM versus LAM in patients with TSC (Box 2). In sporadic cases, LAM formed grossly recognizable, well-demarcated nodules that were primarily concentrated in the outer myometrium and subserosa. The cells were usually spindled but a subset of cases had small amounts of epithelioid cells mixed in. Conversely, LAM occurring in the setting of TSC did not have grossly evident nodules in the uteri but did show microscopic nodules with similar morphology. The cases associated with TSC also showed a more abundant population of epithelioid cells intermixed

with spindled cells that diffusely infiltrated the myometrium in a tongue-like growth pattern. In addition, the involvement of the myometrium was much more diffuse in patients with TSC. Adnexal involvement by LAM was microscopic and showed an appearance similar to the uterine nodules and was present in both sporadic and syndromic cases. Small groups of LAM cells surrounded by lymphatic endothelium have been described as free floating in lymphatic channels. Involvement of pelvic and retroperitoneal lymph nodes is also common but isolated involvement of lymph nodes without uterine or pulmonary LAM is typical of sporadic cases.[27] By immunohistochemistry, LAM is positive for both smooth muscle and melanocytic markers, including desmin, smooth muscle actin, caldesmon, HMB-45, and melan-A.

PERIVASCULAR EPITHELIOID CELL TUMOR

There is abundant morphologic overlap between PEComa and LAM because they are both composed of PECs. Although LAM usually shows small nodules that may or may not be visible grossly, PEComas are mass forming and often have a gross appearance similar to smooth muscle tumors (SMTs). Microscopically, PEComas can be well circumscribed or infiltrative and may be arranged in fascicles, nests, or sheets in a perivascular distribution. There are usually a mixture of spindled and epithelioid cells with clear to eosinophilic granular cytoplasm but may be predominantly epithelioid or spindled (see Fig. 2B). Other common features include pericytomatous vasculature, stromal hyalinization, multinucleated giant cells, spider cells, and tumor cell discohesion.[22,25] PEComas show the same immunophenotype as LAM with

Table 2
Diagnostic criteria for tuberous sclerosis complex

Major Criteria	Minor Criteria
Skin/oral cavity: hypomelanotic macules, angiofibromas, ungual fibromas, shagreen patch	Skin/oral cavity: confetti skin lesions, dental enamel pits, intraoral fibromas
Central nervous system: cortical dysplasias (tubers), subependymal nodules, subependymal giant cell astrocytoma	Multiple renal cysts
Cardiac rhabdomyoma	Retinal achromic patch
Pulmonary LAM	Nonrenal hamartomas
Renal angiomyolipomas	
Multiple retinal hamartomas	

Definitive diagnosis requires 2 major criteria OR 1 major criteria with greater than 2 minor criteria OR the presence a *TSC1* or *TSC2* pathogenic mutation. Possible diagnosis requires either 1 major criteria OR greater than 2 minor criteria.

Adapted from DiMario FJ Jr, Sahin M, Ebrahimi-Fakhari D. Tuberous sclerosis complex. Pediatr Clin North Am 2015;62(3):633–48.

Fig. 2. (*A*) Uterine LAM in a patient with TSC. The proliferation shows spindled and epithelioid-shaped cells arranged in fascicles and oriented around irregularly dilated cleftlike vasculature. Note the tongue-like growth pattern and a few small groups of LAM cells floating within the lymphatic spaces. (*B*) Uterine PEComa. The tumor shows a mixture of spindled and epithelioid cells with clear to eosinophilic cytoplasm and arranged in fascicles. The tumors shows also stromal hyalization and variable nuclear atypia.

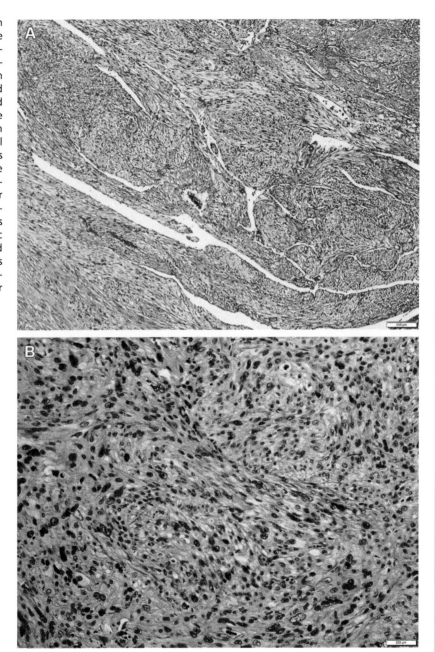

dual expression of smooth muscle and melanocytic markers. In a series of gynecologic PEComas, HMB-45, microphthalmia transcription factor (MiTF), and melan-A were positive in 100%, 92%, and 88% of cases, respectively. The staining pattern of HMB-45 is strong but can be patchy and focal (see Fig. 2C). Melan-A is also only focally positive but with less intensity than HMB-45, necessitating careful inspection to identify immunoreactive cells. Desmin, smooth muscle actin, and h-caldesmon also showed

high sensitivity—they were positive in 100%, 93%, and 92% of cases, respectively.[22]

There exists a subset of PEComas that harbors *TFE3* gene rearrangements with frequent pure epithelioid morphology and a characteristic nested or alveolar growth pattern (see Fig. 2D), which have not been reported as occurring in patients with TSC.[28,29] Because it appears that *TFE3* abnormalities are mutually exclusive with mutations in *TSC1* and *TSC2*, this subset of PEComas is likely not part of the spectrum of TSC.[30]

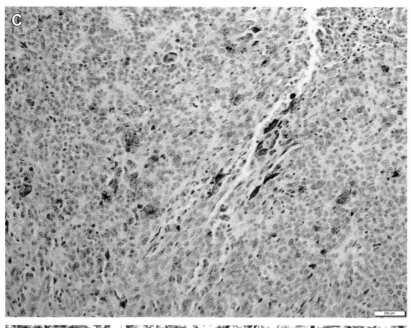

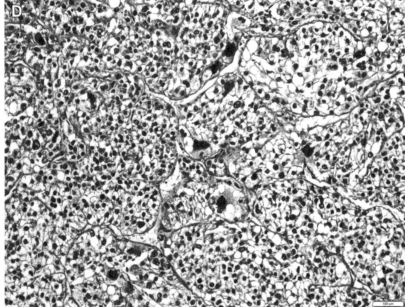

Fig. 2. (continued). (*C*) Immunohistochemistry for HMB-45 in uterine PEComa. The intensity is usually strong but may be only focally positive. (*D*) Uterine PEComa. The tumor shows a nested or alveolar architecture with an epithelioid appearance. Note the focal tumor cell discohesion, spider cells, and staghorn/pericytomatous vasculature. This PEComa belongs to a subset of PEComas with *TFE3* rearrangements, which are likely not related to TSC.

DIFFERENTIAL DIAGNOSIS

The differential diagnosis of LAM includes diffuse leiomyomatosis, intravascular leiomyomatosis, and endometrial stromal sarcoma. Morphologic features in separating LAM from these lesions include the characteristic vasculature as well as the multifocality and microscopic size of the lesions. Confirming melanocytic differentiation with immunohistochemistry can aid in separating LAM

from other SMTs but can be problematic due to the occurrence of HMB-45 immunoreactivity in the latter. Diffuse and strong immunoreactivity for smooth muscle markers, including h-caldesmon, may aid in making the distinction between endometrial stromal sarcoma and LAM.

One of the major entities in the differential diagnosis of PEComa is an SMT, including leiomyoma (Box 3) and leiomyosarcoma. Important morphologic features seen in PEComas that are not

Box 2
Key features of gynecologic lymphangioleiomyomatosis: tuberous sclerosis–related versus sporadic

	Tuberous Sclerosis	Sporadic
Grossly evident uterine nodules	No	Yes
Uterine involvement	Diffuse	Outer myometrium, subserosa
Growth pattern	Infiltrative, tongue-like	Well-circumscribed
Cell shape	Epithelioid/spindled	Predominantly spindled
Adnexal involvement	Yes	Yes
Lymph node involvement	Yes	Yes[a]
Pulmonary involvement	Yes	Yes[a]

[a] Lymph node involvement without uterine or pulmonary involvement is more common in sporadic cases.

frequently seen in SMTs include clear to eosinophilic granular cytoplasm (compared with densely eosinophilic cytoplasm in SMTs), stromal hyalinization, spider cells, and an intimately associated delicate vasculature. Although HMB-45 immunoreactivity has been reported in SMTs, melan-A positivity has been shown more specific for PEComa in this setting.[22]

PROGNOSIS

Uterine PEComas are mostly benign, but malignant behavior has been described. Criteria to predict malignant behavior were proposed by Folpe and colleagues,[31] who found that tumors with a mitotic index of greater than 1 per 50 high-power fields, a size greater than 8 cm, and necrosis were associated with a higher incidence of recurrence and metastatsis. Gynecologic-specific prognostic factors have also been proposed.[22] Schoolmeester and colleagues[22] found that malignant tumors are usually greater than 5 cm, have an infiltrative growth pattern, and show high-grade

nuclear features, necrosis, vascular invasion, and greater 1 per 50 high-power fields. Uterine LAM shows a benign clinical course; however, there is 1 reported case of an angiosarcoma arising in association with LAM in a patient with TSC.[23] The tumor showed lymphatic endothelial differentiation as it was reportedly positive for CD31 and D2-40 but negative for CD34 and factor VIII by immunohistochemistry.[23] Because uterine LAM rarely exists without the presence of pulmonary LAM, the prognosis for these patients largely depends on their lung disease.

COWDEN SYNDROME

Cowden syndrome (CS), one of several disorders under the umbrella term, *PTEN hamartoma tumor syndrome*, is an autosomal dominant syndrome that develops in individuals with pathogenic germline mutations in the *phosphatase and tensin homolog gene* (*PTEN*), a tumor suppressor, located on 10q23.3. Other genes implicated in the syndrome include *SDH-B*, *SDH-C*, *SDH-D*,

Box 3
Key features of uterine PEComa versus typical leiomyoma

	PEComa	Typical Leiomyoma
Cell shape	Spindled/epithelioid	Predominantly spindled
Cytoplasm	Clear to eosinophilic, granular	Densely eosinophilic
Vasculature	Frequently staghorn/pericytomatous	Thick-walled
Stromal hyalinization	Frequent	Rare
Spider cells	Frequent	Rare
Smooth muscle IHC	Positive	Positive
Melanocytic IHC (HMB-45, melan-A)	Frequent	Rare

Abbreviation: IHC, immunohistochemistry.

and *KLLN*.[32] In addition to multiple hamartomas, patients are at risk for many types of malignancies, including endometrial, breast, thyroid, colon, and kidney cancers (Table 3). Although the prevalence of CS is estimated at approximately 1 in 200,000 to 250,000 individuals, the true incidence is difficult to ascertain due to the subtle and variable presentation in many patients, leading to underdiagnosis.[33–37]

CLINICAL FEATURES

Patients with CS have up to a 28% lifetime risk of developing endometrial cancer (EC), which is one of the major criteria for diagnosis.[38,39] The prevalence of CS in unselected EC patients is largely unknown; in a series of 240 consecutive EC patients, no germline pathogenic *PTEN* abnormalities were identified.[40] The age at presentation is also not well determined but in one series of patients with CS, the mean age at diagnosis of EC was 44 years.[32] ECs have also been reported in adolescents as young as 14 years who were subsequently diagnosed with CS.[41–43] In addition to EC, women are prone to developing uterine leiomyomas, benign ovarian cysts, and menstrual abnormalities.[32,44,45] Nonmalignant manifestations of CS include multiple hamartomatous tumors in various organs, especially the gastrointestinal tract; macrocephaly; mucocutaneous lesions (facial tricholemmomas and papillomatous oral lesions); and benign breast or thyroid disease. Significant predictors of germline *PTEN* abnormality in patients with EC include carcinoma diagnosed at age 50 years or less, macrocephaly, and synchronous/metachronous RCC.[32]

PTEN AND ENDOMETRIAL CANCER

Few studies have examined the histologic subtype of ECs in CS. In a large study of 371 patients with CS, endometrioid histology was most common (42%) followed by serous/clear cell (5%) and mucinous (0.3%). In half of the patients, however, the histology was not known.[32] There have also been isolated case reports of cancers with endometrioid histology occurring in patients with CS[41–43,46] (Fig. 3A).

Other evidence that suggests endometrioid histology as the predominant subtype in this syndrome is the high rate of *PTEN* abnormalities in unselected endometrioid EC. The endometrial Cancer Genome Atlas found *PTEN* abnormalities in 77% of nonultramutated endometrioid adenocarcinomas, whereas they were rarely seen in serous carcinomas.[47] Another study found *PTEN* mutations in 67% and 90% of low-grade and high-grade endometrioid tumors, respectively, whereas they were found in only 2.7% of serous cancers.[48] *PTEN* immunohistochemistry appears to be a reliable method in detecting *PTEN* abnormalities in the tumor[49,50] (see Fig. 3B). Unfortunately, there are no other morphologic features described that are specific for the syndrome because large morphologically detailed studies are lacking.

PROGNOSIS

Due to the rarity of the syndrome, there have been no described associations with prognosis and ECs in the setting of CS. Patients with CS, however, have a 7-fold increase risk of a secondary malignancy compared with the general population.[51] Because many of the cancers that have been

Table 3
Diagnostic criteria for Cowden syndrome

Pathognomonic Criteria (Mucocutaneous Lesions)	Major Criteria	Minor Criteria
Facial trichilemmomas	Breast cancer	Thyroid lesions (ie, goiter)
Acral keratoses	Thyroid cancer (especially	Mental retardation
Mucosa/cutaneous papillomatous	follicular type)	Hamartomatous intestinal polyps
	Macrocephaly	Fibrocystic breast disease
	Lhermitte-Duclos disease	Lipomas
	(cerebellar dysplastic	Fibromas
	gangliocytoma)	Renal Cell Cancer
	Endometrial Cancer	Uterine leiomyomas
		Genitourinary malformation

The diagnosis requires the presence of pathognomic mucocutaneous lesions OR 2 major criteria (1 must be macrocephaly or Lhermitte-Duclos) OR 1 major and 3 minor criteria OR 4 minor criteria.
Adapted from Pilarski R, Eng C. Will the real Cowden syndrome please stand up (again)? Expanding mutational and clinical spectra of the PTEN hamartoma tumour syndrome. J Med Genet 2004;41(5):323–6.

Fig. 3. (A) Well-differentiated endometrioid adenocarcinoma in a patient with Cowden Syndrome. (B) Immunohistochemistry for PTEN. Staining is lost, indicative of a genetic abnormality in PTEN.

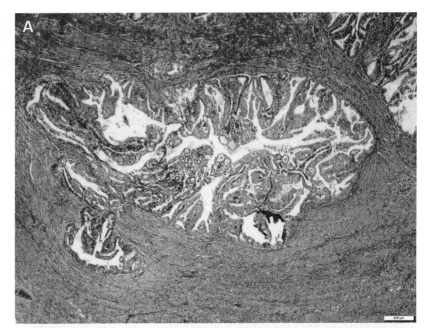

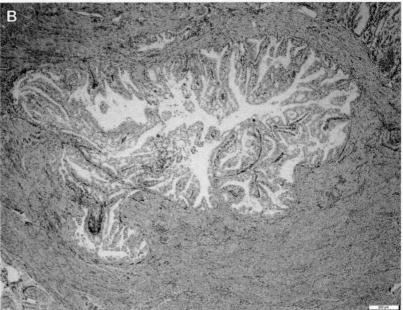

reported in the setting of CS are endometrioid tumors, their prognosis may be similar to that of sporadic endometrioid tumors.

NEVOID BASAL CELL CARCINOMA SYNDROME

Nevoid basal cell carcinoma syndrome (NBCC), also known as Gorlin-Goltz syndrome and as Gorlin syndrome, is an autosomal dominant syndrome that results from a germline heterozygous mutation in 1 of multiple genes, including Patched 1 (PTCH1) gene as well as PTCH2 and SUFU.[52,53] Classic symptoms include early onset of basal cell carcinomas, odontogenic keratocysts, cerebral calcifications, palmar/plantar pits, and spine and rib anomalies (Table 4). Ovarian fibroma is another manifestation that may occur in approximately 17% to 24% of women with NBCC and is 1 of the minor criteria for establishing a diagnosis. Other reported tumors include fibrothecoma, sclerosing stromal tumor, leiomyosarcoma, and fibrosarcoma.[54–57]

Table 4
Diagnostic criteria for NBCC

Major Criteria	Minor Criteria
Odontogenic keratocysts of the jaw	Macrocephaly
Multiple basal cell carcinomas or 1 in patient <20 y	Fused, splayed, or bifid ribs
Palmar/plantar pits	Skeletal abnormalities (Sprengel deformity, pectus deformity, syndactyly, kyphoscoliosis)
Calcifications of the falx cerebri	Craniofacial abnormalities (cleft lip/palate, frontal bossing, hypertelorism)
Medulloblastoma in early childhood	Ovarian or cardiac fibromas
First-degree relative with NBCC	Lymphomesenteric cysts
	Ocular abnormalities (cataracts, glaucoma, developmental defects)

The diagnosis requires 2 major criteria OR 1 major and 2 minor criteria OR 1 major criteria and genetic confirmation.
   Adapted from John AM, Schwartz RA. Basal cell nevus syndrome: an update on genetics and treatment. Br J Dermatol 2015:174(1):68–76.

CLINICAL FEATURES

The mean age of diagnosis of fibromas in NBCC is approximately 30 years compared with sporadic fibromas, which typically present in the fifth and sixth decades.[58,59] They are most frequently bilateral (75%) and calcified. In addition, they may overlap medially, forming a single central calcified mass and may be misdiagnosed as a calcified uterine leiomyoma on imaging studies.[60] Sporadic fibromas, however, are almost always unilateral and show calcifications only 10% of the time. If present, the calcifications are usually focal as opposed to diffuse in patients with NBCC[61] (Box 4). Although patients usually present with extraovarian symptoms, rarely, the fibroma may be the first manifestation of the disease. Usually, patients are asymptomatic but may show symptoms of a mass effect or acute abdomen when large or produce complications, such as ovarian torsion.[62,63] Unusual features include virilization and renin secretion.[57,64,65]

GROSS/MICROSCOPIC FEATURES AND DIAGNOSIS

Gross examination shows a white to tan, firm surface. They frequently have a characteristic multinodular growth pattern (Fig. 4A) and may be multifocal. Large dystrophic calcifications are usually present and can make sectioning difficult (see Fig. 4B). They are less frequently soft, edematous, or cystic but may show hemorrhage and necrosis, especially in larger, cellular tumors.

Microscopically, fibromas in patients with NBCC are similar to those sporadic tumors, with the exception of calcifications. They are composed of ovoid to spindle-type cells with scant cytoplasm that are typically arranged in a fascicular or storiform pattern. The cellularity varies and may show areas of hypocellularity and hypercellularity in the same tumor. There is usually collagen deposition between intervening cells, sometimes forming hyaline plaques. Syndromic fibromas show the same immunophenotype as sporadic fibromas.

DIFFERENTIAL DIAGNOSIS

As discussed previously, fibromas in the setting of NBCC may mimic the appearance of a calcified leiomyoma on imaging as well as grossly and microscopically. Immunohistochemistry for sex-cord stromal markers, such as inhibin, calretinin, and CD56, aid in distinguishing the entities

Box 4
Key features of fibromas associated with nevoid basal cell carcinoma syndrome versus sporadic fibromas

	Nevoid Basal Cell Carcinoma Syndrome	Sporadic fibromas
Laterality	Bilateral	Unilateral
Calcifications	75% of cases/diffuse	10% of cases/focal
Mean age at diagnosis	30 (often in first or second decade)	50
Growth pattern	Multinodular/multifocal	Single mass

Fig. 4. (*A*) Fibroma with characteristic multinodular growth pattern in a child with nevoid basal cell carcinoma syndrome. (*B*) Fibroma with a large, dystrophic calcification in a patient with nevoid basal cell carcinoma syndrome.

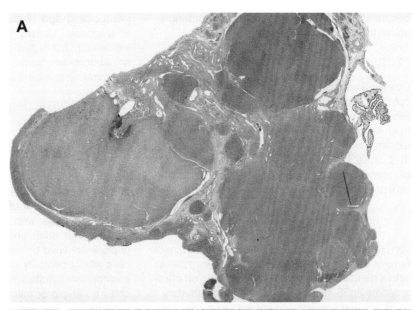

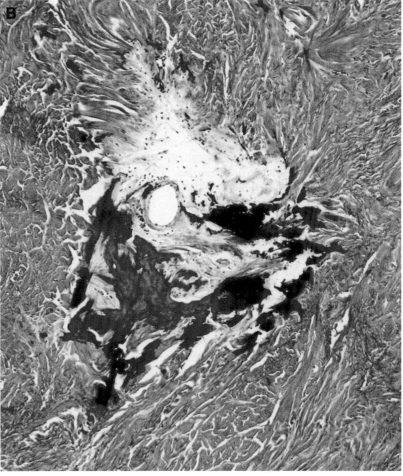

because fibromas may occasionally be immunoreactive for smooth muscle markers.

PROGNOSIS

Ovarian fibromas in patients with NBCC are benign but have been reported to recur.[66] Primary ovarian leiomyosarcoma[54] and fibrosarcoma[55] also have been reported. The prognosis is largely related to extraovarian manifestations and the morbidity they cause. Conservative therapy with preservation of normal ovarian tissue is recommended to prevent premature menopause and to preserve fertility.

VON HIPPEL-LINDAU SYNDROME

von Hippel-Lindau (VHL) is an autosomal dominant familial cancer syndrome that occurs in patients with a germline mutation in the *VHL* gene on chromosome 3p25.3. The incidence is approximately 1 in 36,000 and predisposes patients to a wide variety of benign and malignant tumors, including hemangioblastoma, RCC, pheochromocytoma, and pancreatic lesions[67–69] (Table 5). Clear cell papillary cystadenoma (CCPC) is another tumor that occurs in patients with VHL and is common in men with the syndrome. It usually originates in the epididymis and if bilateral is considered pathognomonic for VHL.[70] It also has been described in women with VHL, usually in the broad ligament or mesosalpinx; however, it is much less common, with only 11 cases reported in the literature.[71–78] A small subset of these tumors has been described as occurring sporadically in patients without VHL.

CLINICAL FEATURES

All but 2 cases of CCPC described in women have been in patients with VHL. Most patients are of childbearing age or perimenopausal at the time of diagnosis. Usually the lesions are discovered incidentally but a few patients had symptoms of an abdominal mass. Most of the tumors are unilateral.[71,72]

GROSS/MICROSCOPIC FEATURES AND DIAGNOSIS

Grossly, the tumors show a thick fibrous capsule and often have adhesions. They have ranged in size from 3 cm to 6.5 cm. They are partially cystic and solid and may show papillary excrescences within a cyst. Microscopically, they form tubulopapillary structures with broad to finely branched papillae that often show a hyalinized core. The papillae are lined by uniform cuboidal to columnar cells with a centrally placed nucleus and clear to eosinophilic cytoplasm (Fig. 5). The cells usually show no atypia or mitotic activity. By immunohistochemistry, the cells are positive for pancytokeratin, CK7, EMA, and PAX2. CD10 and WT1 are often positive whereas RCC, estrogen receptor, and inhibin are usually negative.[71,72,76] Based on the immunophenotype and frequent association with mesonephric duct system, many investigators favor a mesonephric origin.

DIFFERENTIAL DIAGNOSIS

One of the main entities in the differential diagnosis includes ovarian clear cell carcinoma (OCC) due to shared morphologic and immunophenotypic characteristics, including papillae lined by a single layer of cuboidal cells, clear cytoplasm, hyalinized stroma, and immunoreactivity for CK7 and EMA. The nonovarian location and the absence of nuclear atypia, prominent nucleoli, and mitotic activity all favor CCPC. In addition, CCPC lacks the

Table 5	
Diagnostic criteria for von Hippel-Lindau Syndrome	
Patients with No Family History of von Hippel-Lindau (Need 2 or More)	**Patients with Positive Family History (Need 1 or More)**
Hemangioblastomas (multiple) of the retina, spine, or brain	Retinal angioma
Hemangioblastoma (single) with visceral manifestations (multiple kidney or pancreatic cysts)	Spinal or cerebellar hemangioblastoma
Renal cell carcinoma	Adrenal or extra-adrenal pheochromocytoma
Adrenal or extra-adrenal pheochromocytoma	Renal cell carcinoma
Endolymphatic cyst tumors, papillary cystadenomas, or pancreatic neuroendocrine tumors	Multiple renal or pancreatic cysts

For patients with no family history, the diagnosis requires 2 or more of the listed lesions. Patients with a family history need 1 or more of the listed manifestations.

Adapted from Frantzen C, Klasson TD, Links TP, et al. Von Hippel-Lindau syndrome. In: Pagon RA, Adam MP, Ardinger HH, et al, editors. GeneReviews(R). Seattle (WA): 1993.

Fig. 5. CCPC of the broad ligament in a patient VHL. The tumor shows a papillary architecture lined by a monolayer of cuboidal cells with clear to eosinophilic cytoplasm. Note the absence of atypia or mitotic activity. (*Courtesy of* Dr Glenn McCluggage, Royal Group of Hospitals Trust, Northern Ireland, UK.)

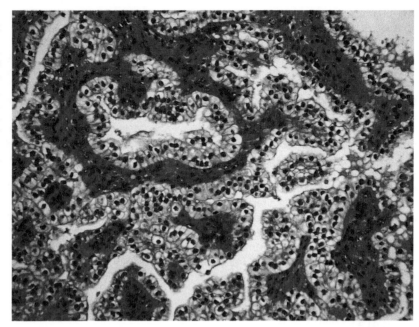

additional characteristic tubulocystic and solid growth patterns seen in OCC. RCC is also in the differential; patients with VHL have a high incidence of renal cancers. Immunohistochemistry for CK7 helps differentiate CCPC from clear cell RCC (**Box 5**).

PROGNOSIS

CCPC is considered a benign entity; however in 1 reported case, a patient presented with advanced-stage disease but without evidence of recurrence after 15 years.[71] In another case, 1 patient had recurrence 5 years after the original diagnosis.[76] Prognosis for these patients is usually related to the malignancies that occur in the syndrome, especially RCC.

MAFFUCCI SYNDROME AND OLLIER DISEASE

Ollier disease (OD) and Maffucci syndrome (MS) are enchondromatoses classified as type I and type II

Box 5
Differential diagnosis of clear cell papillary cystadenoma

	Clear Cell Papillary Cystadenoma	Ovarian Clear Cell Carcinoma	Clear Cell Renal Cell Carcinoma (Metastatic to Adnexa)
Typical location	Broad ligament Mesosalpinx	Ovary	Ovary
Laterality	Unilateral	Unilateral	Variable
Clear cells	Yes	Yes	Yes
Papillary growth pattern	Yes	Yes	Rare pseudopapillary
Nuclear atypia	No	Yes	Yes
Mitotic activity	No	Yes	Yes
Other growth patterns	No	Solid, tubulocystic	Trabecular, tubular, nested, microcystic
Association with VHL	Yes (most cases in females)	No	Yes
Endometriosis associated	No	Yes	No
PAX8+ by IHC	Probably	Yes	Yes
Distinguishing IHC	May be WT1+, usually RCC−	NapsinA+, HNF1β+	CK7−, RCC+

Abbreviations: CCRCC, clear cell RCC; HNF1β, hepatocyte, nuclear factor−1 beta; IHC, immunohistochemistry; PAX8, paired box gene 8; WT1, Wilms tumor 1.

enchondromatosis, respectively. When the disease consists of enchondromatosis only, it is classified as OD; however, when hemangiomas are present, it is known as MS.[79] The estimated incidence of OD is approximately 1 in 100,000 individuals whereas MS is even less frequent.[80] It is characterized by the presence of multiple enchondromas, or benign cartilaginous tumors of bone, which may result in skeletal deformities as well as the development of chondrosarcoma. Although most cases of OD and MS are considered nonfamilial, a small subset of patients with OD inherits the disease in an autosomal dominant fashion. Implicated genes in these syndromes include a receptor for parathyroid hormone and *parathyroid hormone-related protein (PTHR1)*[81] and *IDH1* and *IDH2*.[82] An association between these enchondromatoses and juvenile granulosa cell tumors (JGCTs) of the ovary has been described.[83–88]

CLINICAL FEATURES

Most of the patients who develop JGCTs in the setting of MS/OD do so in the first decade of life and frequently present with precocious puberty due to estrogen production of the tumor.[88] Patients may have symptoms of an abdominal mass, which is usually palpable on pelvic or rectal examination. In other cases, the mass was discovered incidentally during imaging studies for their enchondromatosis. JGCTs are most frequently unilateral and confined to the ovary at presentation.[89]

GROSS/MICROSCOPIC FEATURES AND DIAGNOSIS

JGCTs are mass forming with an average size of 12.5 cm. They may be solid, cystic, or more frequently a combination of both. There is usually abundant hemorrhage. Microscopically, the tumor may form diffuse sheets, nodules, or pseudopapillae of immature-appearing luteinized granulosa cells. In addition, the cells frequently form round to oval follicles containing eosinophilic or basophilic material (**Fig. 6**). Variable quantities of luteinized theca cells also may be present. Cytologically, the cells are mildly atypical but can show marked pleomorphism as well as abundant mitotic activity in some cases. By immunohistochemistry, JGCTs are positive for the typical sex-cord stromal markers, including inhibin and calretinin.

DIFFERENTIAL DIAGNOSIS

The differential diagnosis of JGCT includes the adult variant of granulosa cell tumor, small cell carcinoma of hypercalcemic type (SCCH), and various germ cell tumors. Features that distinguish it from the adult variant of granulosa cell tumor include a low nuclear-to-cytoplasm ratio, follicular spaces, brisk mitotic activity, the absence of nuclear grooves or Call-Exner bodies, and the young age of presentation in most patients. SCCHs occur in young patients and may form follicle-like spaces; however, they are clinically aggressive tumors

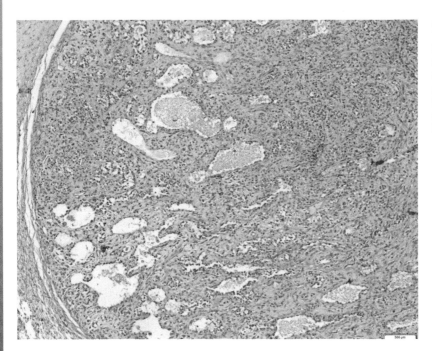

Fig. 6. JGCT of the ovary. The tumor shows granulosa cells forming follicle spaces with eosinophilic material in the lumen. An association between this tumor and enchondromatosis (OD and MS) has been described.

that usually present at advanced stage, lack estrogen production, and are associated with hypercalcemia in most patients. In addition, defects in the gene *SMARCA4* have been implicated in the pathogenesis SCCH, which results in loss of expression of its corresponding protein BRG1, a finding that can be confirmed by immunohistochemistry.[90] Another immunohistochemical marker, FOXL2, which is positive in almost all sex-cord stromal tumors, also may aid in distinguishing SCCH as well as germ cell tumors from JGCTs which are positive for this marker.[91]

PROGNOSIS

In a large series of JGCTs, 92% of patients were alive and free of disease at the time of follow-up.[89] Due to the predominantly indolent course of JGCT, the prognosis of patients with OD/MS is often related to the malignant transformation of enchondromas to chondrosarcoma.

CARNEY COMPLEX

Carney complex (CNC) is an autosomal dominant multiple neoplasia and lentiginosis syndrome, with most cases due to a germline abnormality in the *protein kinase A regulatory subunit-1-alpha* (*PRKAR1A*) gene located on chromosome 17q.[92] It is a rare disease with an unknown prevalence,[93] which predisposes patients to multiple neoplasias, including cardiac, endocrine, cutaneous, and neural myxomatous tumors as well as a variety of pigmented lesions of the skin and mucosa. It also may

be predisposed to a variety of malignant tumors, including cancers of the gastrointestinal tract, thyroid, and breast (Table 6). Its clinical features often overlap with other disorders, including McCune-Albright syndreme, Peutz-Jeghers syndrome, familial multiple endocrine neoplasia, and Cowden Syndrome.[94] Female patients with CNC develop a variety of benign and malignant cysts and tumors involving the ovary.[95]

OVARIAN LESIONS IN CARNEY COMPLEX

In a retrospective analysis of a large group of women with CNC, 2.2% of patients had ovarian tumors that required surgery, including multiple complex cysts, endometrioid adenocarcinoma, and a metastatic mucinous adenocarcinoma. In addition, ovarian lesions were found in 58% of patients with CNC in an autopsy series. These lesions included benign follicular cysts and teratomas.[95] Although these findings are nonspecific, their presence in combination with the reported clinical manifestations may raise the possibility of CNC.

DIFFERENTIAL DIAGNOSIS

Despite overlapping clinical features with Peutz-Jeghers syndrome, such as characteristic spotty skin pigmentation as well as the occurrence of sex-cord stromal cell tumors in men with CNC, none of the ovarian lesions described in Peutz-Jeghers syndrome or the sex-cord stromal tumors that occur in men with CNC seems to be part of the syndrome in women.[95]

Table 6
Diagnostic criteria for Carney complex

Major Criteria	Supplemental Criteria	Minor Criteria
Spotty skin pigmentation	Affected first-degree relative	Intense freckling
Cutaneous/mucosal/cardiac myxoma	Pathogenic variant in *PRKACA, PRKACB*	Café au lait spots
Breast myxomatosis	Pathogenic variant in *PRKAR1A*	Endocrine dysfunction (in the absence of clinical acromegaly)
Primary pigmented nodular adrenocortical disease		Cardiomyopathy
Acromegaly due to growth hormone–producing adenoma		History of Cushing syndrome, acromegaly or sudden death in extended family
Thyroid carcinoma		Pilonidal sinus
Psammomatous melanotic schwannoma		Colon polyps
Blue nevus (multiple)		Multiple skin tags, lipomas
Multiple breast adenomas		Hyperprolactinemia
Osteochondromyxoma		Thyroid nodules
		Family history of thyroid, colon, pancreas, ovary (both benign and malignant)

The diagnosis requires 2 major criteria OR 2 major and 1 supplemental criteria.
Adapted from Correa R, Salpea P, Stratakis CA. Carney complex: an update. Eur J Endocrinol 2015;173(4):M85–97.

PROGNOSIS

Although most of the ovarian lesions in CNC are benign, the prognosis of these patients largely depends on the clinical course of malignancies associated with the syndrome.

REFERENCES

1. Lehtonen HJ. Hereditary leiomyomatosis and renal cell cancer: update on clinical and molecular characteristics. Fam Cancer 2011;10(2):397–411.
2. Launonen V, Vierimaa O, Kiuru M, et al. Inherited susceptibility to uterine leiomyomas and renal cell cancer. Proc Natl Acad Sci U S A 2001;98(6): 3387–92.
3. Smit DL, Mensenkamp AR, Badeloe S, et al. Hereditary leiomyomatosis and renal cell cancer in families referred for fumarate hydratase germline mutation analysis. Clin Genet 2011;79(1):49–59.
4. Reyes C, Karamurzin Y, Frizzell N, et al. Uterine smooth muscle tumors with features suggesting fumarate hydratase aberration: detailed morphologic analysis and correlation with S-(2-succino)-cysteine immunohistochemistry. Mod Pathol 2014; 27(7):1020–7.
5. Chen YB, Brannon AR, Toubaji A, et al. Hereditary leiomyomatosis and renal cell carcinoma syndrome-associated renal cancer: recognition of the syndrome by pathologic features and the utility of detecting aberrant succination by immunohistochemistry. Am J Surg Pathol 2014;38(5):627–37.
6. Lehtonen R, Kiuru M, Vanharanta S, et al. Biallelic inactivation of fumarate hydratase (FH) occurs in nonsyndromic uterine leiomyomas but is rare in other tumors. Am J Pathol 2004;164(1):17–22.
7. Sanz-Ortega J, Vocke C, Stratton P, et al. Morphologic and molecular characteristics of uterine leiomyomas in hereditary leiomyomatosis and renal cancer (HLRCC) syndrome. Am J Surg Pathol 2013;37(1):74–80.
8. Toro JR, Nickerson ML, Wei MH, et al. Mutations in the fumarate hydratase gene cause hereditary leiomyomatosis and renal cell cancer in families in North America. Am J Hum Genet 2003;73(1):95–106.
9. Stewart L, Glenn GM, Stratton P, et al. Association of germline mutations in the fumarate hydratase gene and uterine fibroids in women with hereditary leiomyomatosis and renal cell cancer. Arch Dermatol 2008;144(12):1584–92.
10. Garg K, Tickoo SK, Soslow RA, et al. Morphologic features of uterine leiomyomas associated with hereditary leiomyomatosis and renal cell carcinoma syndrome: a case report. Am J Surg Pathol 2011; 35(8):1235–7.
11. Joseph NM, Solomon DA, Frizzell N, et al. Morphology and Immunohistochemistry for 2SC and FH aid in detection of fumarate hydratase gene aberrations in uterine leiomyomas from young patients. Am J Surg Pathol 2015;39(11):1529–39.
12. Bardella C, El-Bahrawy M, Frizzell N, et al. Aberrant succination of proteins in fumarate hydratase-deficient mice and HLRCC patients is a robust biomarker of mutation status. J Pathol 2011;225(1): 4–11.
13. Lehtonen HJ, Kiuru M, Ylisaukko-Oja SK, et al. Increased risk of cancer in patients with fumarate hydratase germline mutation. J Med Genet 2006; 43(6):523–6.
14. DiMario FJ Jr, Sahin M, Ebrahimi-Fakhari D. Tuberous sclerosis complex. Pediatr Clin North Am 2015;62(3):633–48.
15. Gyure KA, Hart WR, Kennedy AW. Lymphangiomyomatosis of the uterus associated with tuberous sclerosis and malignant neoplasia of the female genital tract: a report of two cases. Int J Gynecol Pathol 1995;14(4):344–51.
16. Liang SX, Pearl M, Liu J, et al. "Malignant" uterine perivascular epithelioid cell tumor, pelvic lymph node lymphangioleiomyomatosis, and gynecological pecomatosis in a patient with tuberous sclerosis: a case report and review of the literature. Int J Gynecol Pathol 2008;27(1):86–90.
17. Fang CL, Lin YH, Chen WY. Microscopic endometrial perivascular epithelioid cell nodules: a case report with the earliest presentation of a uterine perivascular epithelioid cell tumor. Diagn Pathol 2012;7:117.
18. Hayashi T, Kumasaka T, Mitani K, et al. Prevalence of uterine and adnexal involvement in pulmonary lymphangioleiomyomatosis: a clinicopathologic study of 10 patients. Am J Surg Pathol 2011;35(12): 1776–85.
19. Longacre TA, Hendrickson MR, Kapp DS, et al. Lymphangioleiomyomatosis of the uterus simulating high-stage endometrial stromal sarcoma. Gynecol Oncol 1996;63(3):404–10.
20. Torres VE, Björnsson J, King BF, et al. Extrapulmonary lymphangioleiomyomatosis and lymphangiomatous cysts in tuberous sclerosis complex. Mayo Clin Proc 1995;70(7):641–8.
21. Fadare O, Parkash V, Yilmaz Y, et al. Perivascular epithelioid cell tumor (PEComa) of the uterine cervix associated with intraabdominal "PEComatosis": a clinicopathological study with comparative genomic hybridization analysis. World J Surg Oncol 2004;2:35.
22. Schoolmeester JK, Howitt BE, Hirsch MS, et al. Perivascular epithelioid cell neoplasm (PEComa) of the gynecologic tract: clinicopathologic and immunohistochemical characterization of 16 cases. Am J Surg Pathol 2014;38(2):176–88.
23. Hayashi T, Parkash V, Yilmaz Y, et al. Uterine angiosarcoma associated with lymphangioleiomyomatosis in a patient with tuberous sclerosis complex: an

autopsy case report with immunohistochemical and genetic analysis. Hum Pathol 2012;43(10):1777–84.

24. Matsui K, Tatsuguchi A, Valencia J, et al. Extrapulmonary lymphangioleiomyomatosis (LAM): clinicopathologic features in 22 cases. Hum Pathol 2000; 31(10):1242–8.

25. Lim GS, Oliva E. The morphologic spectrum of uterine PEC-cell associated tumors in a patient with tuberous sclerosis. Int J Gynecol Pathol 2011;30(2): 121–8.

26. Vang R, Kempson RL. Perivascular epithelioid cell tumor ('PEComa') of the uterus: a subset of HMB-45-positive epithelioid mesenchymal neoplasms with an uncertain relationship to pure smooth muscle tumors. Am J Surg Pathol 2002;26(1):1–13.

27. Schoolmeester JK, Park KJ. Incidental nodal lymphangioleiomyomatosis is not a harbinger of pulmonary lymphangioleiomyomatosis: a study of 19 cases with evaluation of diagnostic immunohistochemistry. Am J Surg Pathol 2015;39(10):1404–10.

28. Argani P, Aulmann S, Illei PB, et al. A distinctive subset of PEComas harbors TFE3 gene fusions. Am J Surg Pathol 2010;34(10):1395–406.

29. Schoolmeester JK, Dao LN, Sukov WR, et al. TFE3 translocation-associated perivascular epithelioid cell neoplasm (PEComa) of the gynecologic tract: morphology, immunophenotype, differential diagnosis. Am J Surg Pathol 2015;39(3):394–404.

30. Agaram NP, Sung YS, Zhang L, et al. Dichotomy of genetic abnormalities in PEComas with therapeutic implications. Am J Surg Pathol 2015;39(6): 813–25.

31. Folpe AL, Mentzel T, Lehr HA, et al. Perivascular epithelioid cell neoplasms of soft tissue and gynecologic origin: a clinicopathologic study of 26 cases and review of the literature. Am J Surg Pathol 2005;29(12):1558–75.

32. Mahdi H, Mester JL, Nizialek EA, et al. Germline PTEN, SDHB-D, and KLLN alterations in endometrial cancer patients with Cowden and Cowden-like syndromes: an international, multicenter, prospective study. Cancer 2015;121(5):688–96.

33. Stadler ZK, Robson ME. Inherited predisposition to endometrial cancer: moving beyond Lynch syndrome. Cancer 2015;121(5):644–7.

34. Wong A, Ngeow J. Hereditary syndromes manifesting as endometrial carcinoma: how can pathological features aid risk assessment? Biomed Res Int 2015; 2015:219012.

35. Eng C. Will the real Cowden syndrome please stand up: revised diagnostic criteria. J Med Genet 2000; 37(11):828–30.

36. Haibach H, Burns TW, Carlson HE, et al. Multiple hamartoma syndrome (Cowden's disease) associated with renal cell carcinoma and primary neuroendocrine carcinoma of the skin (Merkel cell carcinoma). Am J Clin Pathol 1992;97(5):705–12.

37. Schrager CA, Schneider D, Gruener AC, et al. Clinical and pathological features of breast disease in Cowden's syndrome: an underrecognized syndrome with an increased risk of breast cancer. Hum Pathol 1998;29(1):47–53.

38. Tan MH, Mester JL, Ngeow J, et al. Lifetime cancer risks in individuals with germline PTEN mutations. Clin Cancer Res 2012;18(2):400–7.

39. Pilarski R, Eng C. Will the real Cowden syndrome please stand up (again)? Expanding mutational and clinical spectra of the PTEN hamartoma tumour syndrome. J Med Genet 2004;41(5):323–6.

40. Black D, Bogomolniy F, Robson ME, et al. Evaluation of germline PTEN mutations in endometrial cancer patients. Gynecol Oncol 2005;96(1):21–4.

41. Baker WD, Soisson AP, Dodson MK. Endometrial cancer in a 14-year-old girl with Cowden syndrome: a case report. J Obstet Gynaecol Res 2013;39(4): 876–8.

42. Elnaggar AC, Spunt SL, Smith W, et al. Endometrial cancer in a 15-year-old girl: a complication of Cowden syndrome. Gynecol Oncol Case Rep 2012;3: 18–9.

43. Schmeler KM, Daniels MS, Brandt AC, et al. Endometrial cancer in an adolescent: a possible manifestation of Cowden syndrome. Obstet Gynecol 2009; 114(2 Pt 2):477–9.

44. Salem OS, Steck WD. Cowden's disease (multiple hamartoma and neoplasia syndrome). A case report and review of the English literature. J Am Acad Dermatol 1983;8(5):686–96.

45. Tan MH, Mester J, Peterson C, et al. A clinical scoring system for selection of patients for PTEN mutation testing is proposed on the basis of a prospective study of 3042 probands. Am J Hum Genet 2011;88(1):42–56.

46. Edwards JM, Alsop S, Modesitt SC. Coexisting atypical polypoid adenomyoma and endometrioid endometrial carcinoma in a young woman with Cowden syndrome: case report and implications for screening and prevention. Gynecol Oncol Case Rep 2012;2(2):29–31.

47. Cancer Genome Atlas Research Network, Kandoth C, Schultz N, et al. Integrated genomic characterization of endometrial carcinoma. Nature 2013; 497(7447):67–73.

48. McConechy MK, Ding J, Cheang MC, et al. Use of mutation profiles to refine the classification of endometrial carcinomas. J Pathol 2012;228(1):20–30.

49. Djordjevic B, Hennessy BT, Li J, et al. Clinical assessment of PTEN loss in endometrial carcinoma: immunohistochemistry outperforms gene sequencing. Mod Pathol 2012;25(5):699–708.

50. Garg K, Broaddus RR, Soslow RA, et al. Pathologic scoring of PTEN immunohistochemistry in endometrial carcinoma is highly reproducible. Int J Gynecol Pathol 2012;31(1):48–56.

51. Ngeow J, Stanuch K, Mester JL, et al. Second malignant neoplasms in patients with Cowden syndrome with underlying germline PTEN mutations. J Clin Oncol 2014;32(17):1818–24.

52. Smith MJ, Beetz C, Williams SG, et al. Germline mutations in SUFU cause Gorlin syndrome-associated childhood medulloblastoma and redefine the risk associated with PTCH1 mutations. J Clin Oncol 2014;32(36):4155–61.

53. John AM, Schwartz RA. Basal cell nevus syndrome: an update on genetics and treatment. Br J Dermatol 2015;174(1):68–76.

54. Seracchioli R, Colombo FM, Bagnoli A, et al. Primary ovarian leiomyosarcoma as a new component in the nevoid basal cell carcinoma syndrome: a case report. Am J Obstet Gynecol 2003;188(4):1093–5.

55. Kraemer BB, Silva EG, Sneige N. Fibrosarcoma of ovary. A new component in the nevoid basal-cell carcinoma syndrome. Am J Surg Pathol 1984;8(3): 231–6.

56. Grechi G, Clemente N, Tozzi A, et al. Laparoscopic treatment of sclerosing stromal tumor of the ovary in a woman with gorlin-goltz syndrome: a case report and review of the literature. J Minim Invasive Gynecol 2015;22(5):892–5.

57. Fox R, Eckford S, Hirschowitz L, et al. Refractory gestational hypertension due to a renin-secreting ovarian fibrothecoma associated with Gorlin's syndrome. Br J Obstet Gynaecol 1994;101(11):1015–7.

58. Kimonis VE, Goldstein AM, Pastakia B, et al. Clinical manifestations in 105 persons with nevoid basal cell carcinoma syndrome. Am J Med Genet 1997;69(3): 299–308.

59. Evans DG, Ladusans EJ, Rimmer S, et al. Complications of the naevoid basal cell carcinoma syndrome: results of a population based study. J Med Genet 1993;30(6):460–4.

60. Gorlin RJ. Nevoid basal-cell carcinoma syndrome. Medicine (Baltimore) 1987;66(2):98–113.

61. Gorlin RJ. Nevoid basal cell carcinoma (Gorlin) syndrome. Genet Med 2004;6(6):530–9.

62. Johnson AD, Hebert AA, Esterly NB. Nevoid basal cell carcinoma syndrome: bilateral ovarian fibromas in a 3 1/2-year-old girl. J Am Acad Dermatol 1986; 14(2 Pt 2):371–4.

63. Raggio M, Kaplan AL, Harberg JF. Recurrent ovarian fibromas with basal cell nevus syndrome (Gorlin syndrome). Obstet Gynecol 1983;61(3 Suppl): 95S–6S.

64. Ismail SM, Walker SM. Bilateral virilizing sclerosing stromal tumours of the ovary in a pregnant woman with Gorlin's syndrome: implications for pathogenesis of ovarian stromal neoplasms. Histopathology 1990;17(2):159–63.

65. Yoshizumi J, Vaughan RS, Jasani B. Pregnancy associated with Gorlin's syndrome. Anaesthesia 1990;45(12):1046–8.

66. Seracchioli R, Bagnoli A, Colombo FM, et al. Conservative treatment of recurrent ovarian fibromas in a young patient affected by Gorlin syndrome. Hum Reprod 2001;16(6):1261–3.

67. Maher ER, Neumann HP, Richard S. von Hippel-Lindau disease: a clinical and scientific review. Eur J Hum Genet 2011;19(6):617–23.

68. Lonser RR, Glenn GM, Walther M, et al. Von Hippel-Lindau disease. Lancet 2003;361(9374):2059–67.

69. Frantzen C, Klasson TD, Links TP, et al. Von Hippel-Lindau syndrome. In: Pagon RA, Adam MP, Ardinger HH, et al, editors. GeneReviews(R). Seattle (WA): 1993.

70. Wernert N, Goebbels R, Prediger L. Papillary cystadenoma of the epididymis. Case report and review of the literature. Pathol Res Pract 1986;181(2): 260–4.

71. Nogales FF, Goyenaga P, Preda O, et al. An analysis of five clear cell papillary cystadenomas of mesosalpinx and broad ligament: four associated with von Hippel-Lindau disease and one aggressive sporadic type. Histopathology 2012;60(5):748–57.

72. Brady A, Nayar A, Cross P, et al. A detailed immunohistochemical analysis of 2 cases of papillary cystadenoma of the broad ligament: an extremely rare neoplasm characteristic of patients with von hippel-lindau disease. Int J Gynecol Pathol 2012; 31(2):133–40.

73. Funk KC, Heiken JP. Papillary cystadenoma of the broad ligament in a patient with von Hippel-Lindau disease. AJR Am J Roentgenol 1989;153(3):527–8.

74. Gaffey MJ, Mills SE, Boyd JC. Aggressive papillary tumor of middle ear/temporal bone and adnexal papillary cystadenoma. Manifestations of von Hippel-Lindau disease. Am J Surg Pathol 1994; 18(12):1254–60.

75. Werness BA, Guccion JG. Tumor of the broad ligament in von Hippel-Lindau disease of probable mullerian origin. Int J Gynecol Pathol 1997;16(3): 282–5.

76. Aydin H, Young RH, Ronnett BM, et al. Clear cell papillary cystadenoma of the epididymis and mesosalpinx: immunohistochemical differentiation from metastatic clear cell renal cell carcinoma. Am J Surg Pathol 2005;29(4):520–3.

77. Gersell DJ, King TC. Papillary cystadenoma of the mesosalpinx in von Hippel-Lindau disease. Am J Surg Pathol 1988;12(2):145–9.

78. Zanotelli DB, Bruder E, Wight E, et al. Bilateral papillary cystadenoma of the mesosalpinx: a rare manifestation of Von Hippel-Lindau disease. Arch Gynecol Obstet 2010;282(3):343–6.

79. Velasco-Oses A, Alonso-Alvaro A, Blanco-Pozo A, et al. Ollier's disease associated with ovarian juvenile granulosa cell tumor. Cancer 1988;62(1):222–5.

80. Silve C, Juppner H. Ollier disease. Orphanet J Rare Dis 2006;1:37.

81. Hopyan S, Gokgoz N, Poon R, et al. A mutant PTH/PTHrP type I receptor in enchondromatosis. Nat Genet 2002;30(3):306–10.

82. Pansuriya TC, van Eijk R, d'Adamo P, et al. Somatic mosaic IDH1 and IDH2 mutations are associated with enchondroma and spindle cell hemangioma in Ollier disease and Maffucci syndrome. Nat Genet 2011;43(12):1256–61.

83. Yuan JQ, Lin XN, Xu JY, et al. Ovarian juvenile granulosa cell tumor associated with Maffucci's syndrome: case report. Chin Med J (Engl) 2004; 117(10):1592–4.

84. Hachi H, Othmany A, Douayri A, et al. Association of ovarian juvenile granulosa cell tumor with Maffucci's syndrome. Gynecol Obstet Fertil 2002;30(9):692–5, [in French].

85. Gell JS, Stannard MW, Ramnani DM, et al. Juvenile granulosa cell tumor in a 13-year-old girl with enchondromatosis (Ollier's disease): a case report. J Pediatr Adolesc Gynecol 1998;11(3):147–50.

86. Tanaka Y, Sasaki Y, Nishihira H, et al. Ovarian juvenile granulosa cell tumor associated with Maffucci's syndrome. Am J Clin Pathol 1992;97(4):523–7.

87. Asirvatham R, Rooney RJ, Watts HG. Ollier's disease with secondary chondrosarcoma associated with ovarian tumour. A case report. Int Orthop 1991; 15(4):393–5.

88. Rietveld L, Nieboer TE, Kluivers KB, et al. First case of juvenile granulosa cell tumor in an adult with Ollier disease. Int J Gynecol Pathol 2009;28(5):464–7.

89. Young RH, Dickersin GR, Scully RE. Juvenile granulosa cell tumor of the ovary. A clinicopathological analysis of 125 cases. Am J Surg Pathol 1984;8(8): 575–96.

90. Karanian-Philippe M, Velasco V, Longy M, et al. SMARCA4 (BRG1) loss of expression is a useful marker for the diagnosis of ovarian small cell carcinoma of the hypercalcemic type (ovarian rhabdoid tumor): a comprehensive analysis of 116 rare gynecologic tumors, 9 soft tissue tumors, and 9 melanomas. Am J Surg Pathol 2015;39(9):1197–205.

91. Al-Agha OM, Huwait HF, Chow C, et al. FOXL2 is a sensitive and specific marker for sex cord-stromal tumors of the ovary. Am J Surg Pathol 2011;35(4): 484–94.

92. Kirschner LS, Sandrini F, Monbo J, et al. Genetic heterogeneity and spectrum of mutations of the PRKAR1A gene in patients with the carney complex. Hum Mol Genet 2000;9(20):3037–46.

93. Correa R, Salpea P, Stratakis CA. Carney complex: an update. Eur J Endocrinol 2015;173(4):M85–97.

94. Stratakis CA, Carney JA, Lin JP, et al. Carney complex, a familial multiple neoplasia and lentiginosis syndrome. Analysis of 11 kindreds and linkage to the short arm of chromosome 2. J Clin Invest 1996; 97(3):699–705.

95. Stratakis CA, Papageorgiou T, Premkumar A, et al. Ovarian lesions in carney complex: clinical genetics and possible predisposition to malignancy. J Clin Endocrinol Metab 2000;85(11):4359–66.

Laboratory Assays in Evaluation of Lynch Syndrome in Patients with Endometrial Carcinoma

Bojana Djordjevic, MD[a],*, Russell R. Broaddus, MD, PhD[b]

KEYWORDS

• Lynch syndrome • Endometrial cancer • Molecular diagnostic testing

Key points

• Immunohistochemistry, microsatellite instability analysis, and MLH1 promoter methylation analysis constitute the cornerstone of laboratory molecular testing of endometrial tumors for Lynch syndrome.

• Discrepancies between genetic, immunohistochemistry, and microsatellite instability analyses may arise and can often be explained as a reflection of the underlying tumor biology.

• Although universal endometrial tumor screening is recommended in order to identify the most patients with possible Lynch syndrome, the current practice of screening is highly variable across different centers and countries.

• Lynch syndrome–associated endometrial tumors are associated with several pathologic characteristics that may be used by pathologists to trigger tissue testing.

ABSTRACT

This article reviews the main tissue testing modalities for Lynch Syndrome in the pathology laboratory, such as immunohistochemistry and PCR based analyses, and discusses their routine application, interpretation pitfalls, and troubleshooting of common technical performance issues. Discrepancies between laboratory and genetic testing may arise, and are examined in the context of the complexity of molecular abnormalities associated with Lynch Syndrome. The merits of targeted versus universal screening in a changing healthcare climate are addressed. In the absence of comprehensive screening programs, specific tumor topography and histological features that may prompt pathologist-initiated molecular tumor testing are outlined.

LYNCH SYNDROME

Lynch Syndrome occurs due to a germline mutation in a gene corresponding to a family of DNA mismatch repair (MMR) proteins, Mut L homolog 1 (MLH1), MutS protein homolog 2 (MSH2), MutS homolog 6 (MSH6) and PMS1 Homolog 2, Mismatch Repair System Component (PMS2). The hallmark cancers for Lynch syndrome are colorectal adenocarcinoma and endometrial carcinoma, whereas less common cancer types include ovarian carcinoma, urothelial carcinomas of the ureter/renal pelvis, duodenal adenocarcinoma, and gastric adenocarcinoma. Loss of DNA MMR protein function typically results in high levels of DNA microsatellite instability (MSI). In 15% to 20% of all sporadic endometrial carcinomas, MLH1 immunohistochemical loss and MSI result

Disclosure: The authors have nothing to disclose.
[a] Department of Pathology and Laboratory Medicine, University of Ottawa, The Ottawa Hospital, Eastern Ontario Regional Laboratory, 501 Smyth Road, Ottawa, Ontario K1H 8L6, Canada; [b] Department of Pathology, Unit 85, University of Texas M.D. Anderson Cancer Center, 1515 Holcombe Blvd., Houston, TX 77030, USA
* Corresponding author.
E-mail addresses: bdjordjevic@toh.on.ca; bojanadjordjevicmd@gmail.com

Surgical Pathology 9 (2016) 289–299
http://dx.doi.org/10.1016/j.path.2016.01.007
1875-9181/16/$ – see front matter © 2016 Elsevier Inc. All rights reserved.

from *MLH1* gene promoter methylation with subsequent transcriptional silencing.[1–5]

For most hereditary cancer syndromes, affected individuals are identified from recognition of a constellation of clinical features, such as young age of cancer onset and a strong family history of characteristic cancers, with subsequent germline sequencing of the suspected affected gene. However, tumor tissue testing in the pathology laboratory is a key component of Lynch syndrome diagnosis, involving MMR immunohistochemistry, MSI analysis, and *MLH1* methylation analysis.

TUMOR TESTING AND PITFALLS IN TEST INTERPRETATION

Immunohistochemistry

Immunohistochemistry for MMR proteins is performed using commercially available antibodies that work fairly reliably. Gene mutation of *MMR* genes or methylation of the *MLH1* gene promoter typically results in loss of immunohistochemical expression of the corresponding protein. Complete absence of nuclear expression should be observed in order for a tumor to be considered as having a loss of an MMR marker. Strong nuclear staining in the surrounding endometrial stroma, myometrium, lymphocytes, or normal endometrium should serve as an internal positive control (**Fig. 1**). The MSH2 and MSH6 proteins, and the MLH1 and PMS2 proteins, act as functional pairs.[6] Therefore, when MLH1 protein expression is lost (because of mutation of the *MLH1* gene or methylation of *MLH1* gene promoter), typically there is secondary loss of PMS2 protein expression. Mutation of the PMS2 gene is associated with loss of PMS2 protein but retained MLH1 immunohistochemical expression. Similarly, mutation of the *MSH2* gene typically results in immunohistochemical loss of MSH2 and MSH6 proteins. In contrast, mutation of *MSH6* gene results only in MSH6 protein loss, whereas MSH2 protein expression remains intact.

Regarding MMR immunohistochemistry reporting recommendations, note that, for most cases, the percentage or intensity of staining is not relevant, and the interpretation result should be either positive or negative. Terminology such as "focally positive," "patchy staining," "weakly positive," "positive in x% of cells," or "equivocal staining" should be avoided. If tumor staining is negative, it should be indicated that internal control stromal cells/normal endometrium are positive.

Several pitfalls in the interpretation of MMR immunohistochemistry exist (**Fig. 2**). Most commonly, false-negative nuclear tumor staining occurs in the setting of an inadequate internal positive control. In contrast, immunohistochemical staining of the tumor cells may be focal or weak. In most cases, this represents genuine nuclear staining. Both of these problems may be resolved by repeating the immunohistochemistry with consideration of prolonging the antigen exposure time or using a different tissue block from the same specimen. Another immunohistochemical issue involves cytoplasmic tumor staining, regardless of the presence or the absence of nuclear staining, especially when the tissue has previously been frozen for the purposes of intraoperative consultation. Cytoplasmic staining should be disregarded in the evaluation of MMR immunohistochemistry. In addition, endometrial stroma or tumor-infiltrating lymphocytes may cause

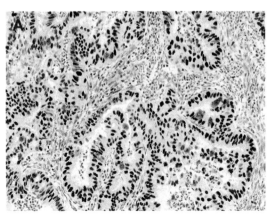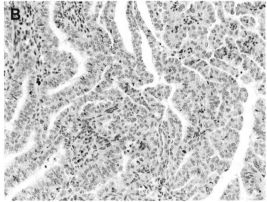

Fig. 1. Application of immunohistochemistry in endometrial carcinoma tissue testing for Lynch syndrome. (*A*) Nuclear expression of mismatch repair proteins (PMS2, 20×). (*B*) Good internal positive control in the surrounding endometrial stroma ensures that the interpretation of mismatch repair protein expression loss is accurate (MSH2, 20×).

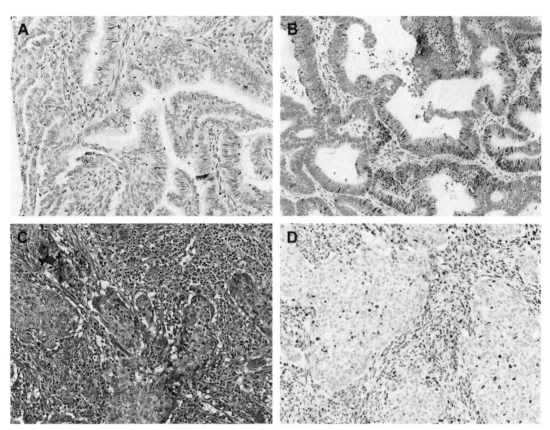

Fig. 2. Common pitfalls in the interpretation of mismatch protein repair immunohistochemistry. (A) Absence of mismatch expression in both the epithelium and the stroma suggests that the immunohistochemical reaction did not work and should be repeated under different conditions or on a different block (MSH6, 20×). (B) Cytoplasmic tumor staining should be disregarded (MSH2, 20×). (C) Some Lynch-associated endometrial tumors show tumor-infiltrating lymphocytes (H&E, 20×). (D) Tumor-infiltrating lymphocytes mimic tumor cells with retained mismatch repair protein expression, which appear within otherwise immunonegative islands of tumor (MLH1, 20×).

difficulties in MMR immunohistochemistry interpretation. However, these cells are typically focal and appear within a background of immunohistochemically negative nests and sheets of tumor cells. Awareness of this pattern and correlation with the corresponding hematoxylin-eosin section should resolve this diagnostic dilemma.

Recently, a heterogeneous pattern of MSH6 expression was described in rare (0.17%) cases of colorectal, endometrial, and sebaceous tumors.[7] Areas of strong MSH6 expression were juxtaposed with areas of complete loss of expression. In some of these cases, MSH2 expression was subtly diminished as well. The cases showed somatic instability within the C8 repeat region of the MSH6 gene along with a normal MSH6 in the germline. In addition, some of the cases showed MLH1/PMS2 loss without evidence of MLH1 promoter methylation. Therefore, heterogeneous expression of MSH6 is not a typical feature of Lynch syndrome, but it does not exclude the

possibility of germline mutations in other MMR genes. The authors have noted similar heterogeneity of MLH1/PMS2 immunohistochemistry, but at this time there is inadequate follow-up information regarding the outcomes of these cases (Fig. 3).

Microsatellite Instability and MLH1 Methylation Analyses

Microsatellites are sequences of DNA composed of repeating units of 1 to 6 base pairs in length. MSI arises as a result of uncorrected errors in DNA replication caused by faulty MMR protein function. MSI analysis is a PCR-based test that requires DNA from both the endometrial tumor and normal nontumor tissues, such as histologically normal cervix, myometrium, or ovary. Appropriate areas of tumor and nontumor tissue are typically circled on a slide by a pathologist, and DNA from tissue in the corresponding paraffin blocks is

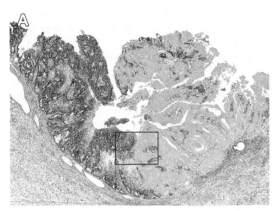
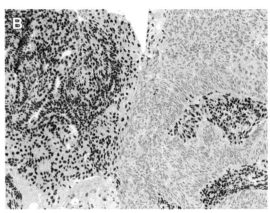

Fig. 3. Heterogeneous pattern of MLH1 mismatch repair protein expression. (*A*) Low power (1×), (*B*) high power (15×) view of the area marked in (*A*). Geographic areas of retained expression are present adjacent to geographic areas of expression loss.

extracted. A panel of 7 markers recommended by the National Cancer Institute[8] (BAT25, BAT26, BAT40, D2S123, D5S346, D173250, and transforming growth factor-βR2) is used to detect changes in the number of microsatellite repeats in the tumor compared with normal tissue (**Fig. 4**). Tumors with an allelic shift in 3 or more microsatellites in the panel are considered MSI high, whereas tumors with no allelic shift in all 7 microsatellites are designated as microsatellite stable (MSS). Tumors with allelic shift in only 1 or 2 microsatellites are considered MSI low.

For MSI-high tumors with loss of MLH1 protein by immunohistochemistry, a polymerase chain reaction (PCR)–based *MLH1* promoter methylation analysis should be performed (**Fig. 5**). In this assay, extracted tissue DNA (typically from the sample used in the MSI assay) is exposed to a bisulfite compound, which converts unmethylated cytosines to uracil, whereas methylated cytosines are resistant to this conversion, which in turn allows the design of different PCR primers that can distinguish between the two types of sequences. *MLH1* promoter methylation and gene silencing is the primary cause of MSI in sporadic endometrial cancers.[9]

Although immunohistochemistry on a specific tissue block may not work well because of suboptimal fixation or tissue processing, MSI and *MLH1* methylation analyses are typically not affected as much and can still yield excellent results. The most common problem involving these analyses is an insufficient amount of tumor in the specimen, so that MSI or *MLH1* promoter methylation is not detected. By recording the approximate amount of tumor present in a section submitted for molecular testing, cases at risk for a false-negative result of this type may be identified in advance. In

instances of tumor heterogeneity or a significant amount of nontumor tissue accompanying tumor tissue in the material submitted for analysis, detection of the molecular abnormality is generally interpreted as evidence of this abnormality being associated with the tumor. Amplification errors in MSI analysis are uncommon. In a large study of colorectal, endometrial, and other Lynch syndrome–associated tumors,[10] only 0.6% of microsatellites amplified suboptimally, with failure at no more than 1 microsatellite per tumor. In only a few of these cases would successful amplification of the missing microsatellite have led to reclassification of the MSI analysis result (ie, MSS to MSI low, or MSI low to MSI high).

DISCREPANCIES BETWEEN TISSUE TESTING AND GENETIC TESTING

Known Mismatch Repair Gene Mutations and Ambiguous or Normal Tissue Testing Results

In some patients with known mutations in the *MMR* genes, the results of MSI analysis and/or MMR immunohistochemistry may be conflicting. For example, full-length but nonfunctional MMR proteins resulting from missense mutations in *MMR* genes may yield MSI-high tumors with intact expression of MMR proteins by immunohistochemistry. Tumors of other patients with known *MMR* gene mutations may have MMR loss by immunohistochemistry, but be MSI low or even MSS. Compared with colorectal carcinoma, endometrial tumors show a lower proportion of unstable microsatellite markers (0.27 for endometrium vs 0.45 for colon per average tumor), have shorter allelic shifts in BAT loci, and a greater proportion of tumors that are MSS (23% of endometrial vs 11% of colon cancer cases).[11] In particular,

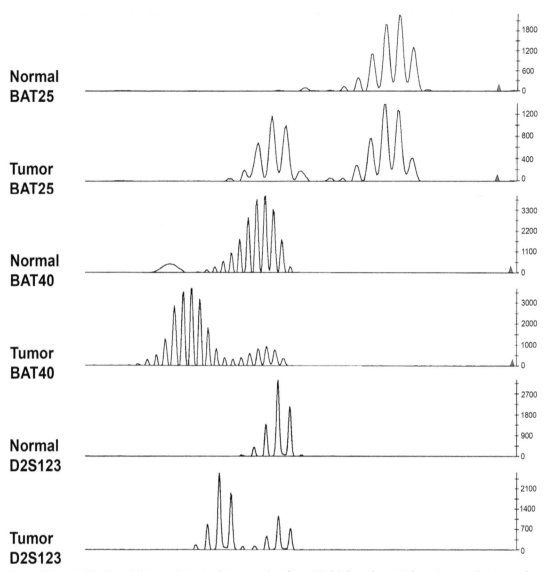

Fig. 4. Microsatellite instability analysis. In this example of an MSI-high endometrial carcinoma, the tumor has allelic shift for the mononucleotide microsatellites BAT25 and BAT40 and the dinucleotide microsatellite D2S123. There are extra peaks in the tumor tracings compared with that of normal tissue for each of the microsatellites.

patients with *MSH6* germline mutations tend to have tumors that are disproportionately MSI low or MSS.[12–14] Furthermore, MSI analysis of paired synchronous ovarian and endometrial carcinomas revealed differing patterns of microsatellite allelic shift, despite the ovarian and endometrial tumors in each pair having lost expression of the same DNA MMR protein by immunohistochemistry.[15] It has been suggested that target genes of MSI are tissue specific, and that this may be the source for differing patterns of MSI across different tumor types.[16] From a tissue testing perspective, these biological phenomena may generate discrepancies

between immunohistochemistry, MSI analysis, and mutation status, particularly when noncolorectal tumors are concerned.

Abnormal Tissue Testing Results and No Detectable Mismatch Repair Gene Mutations

Cases may occur in which MSI and MMR immunohistochemistry are both suggestive of Lynch syndrome, but the genetic analysis does not reveal a pathologic mutation in the *MMR* genes. Several population-based studies using tumor tissue testing methods, including immunohistochemistry

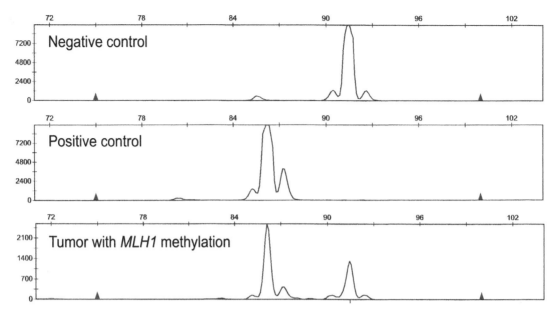

Fig. 5. *MLH1* promoter methylation analysis. In this assay, tumor DNA is treated with bisulfite, which converts cytosine to uracil; methylated cytosines are resistant to such conversion, allowing the creation of different PCR reaction primers, which can differentiate the 2 types of sequences. Tumor DNA is analyzed concurrently with DNA from control cell lines. First tracing, negative control K562 with no *MLH1* methylation; second tracing, positive control RKO with presence of *MLH1* methylation. The endometrial carcinoma in the third tracing has both unmethylated and methylated *MLH1*. The unmethylated peak is likely caused by the presence of contaminating normal stromal cells.

and MSI analysis, have shown that the proportion of patients with endometrial cancers identified as having possible Lynch syndrome is as high as 6% to 10%.[17–19] This percentage is significantly higher than the value of 1% to 2%, which represents the proportion of patients with detected germline mutations.[4,20,21]

Although there are *MMR* gene variants of undetermined significance, which may in the future be reclassified as pathologic mutations with accumulation of experience, there are several other explanations for discrepancies between tissue and genetic testing results that have come to light from recent studies. For example, 5% and 20% to 25% of cases with MSH2/MSH6 immunohistochemical expression defects and a nondetectable germline mutation in the *MSH2* and *MSH6* genes can be accounted for by the presence of *MSH2* inversions (exons 1–7) and epithelial cell adhesion molecule (EPCAM) germline mutations, respectively.[22,23] In the latter instance, mutations in the 3' end of the EPCAM gene, which is located upstream of the MSH2 gene, results in hypermethylation of the *MSH2* promoter and thus transcriptional silencing of an otherwise normal *MSH2* gene.[23] Biallelic somatic (tumor) DNA mutations in MMR genes have also recently been uncovered in 52% to 69% of colorectal and endometrial tumors

suspected for Lynch syndrome based on tissue testing but without detectable germline mutations.[24–26] One of these studies found that most somatic mutations were not the same as typical germline mutations, all tumors had a hypermutator phenotype (>12 mutations/Mb), and 23% of the cases had associated mutations in the catalytic subunit of the DNA polymerase epsilon (*POLE*) gene.[25] It is not clear at this time whether the *POLE* gene mutations precede the *MMR* gene mutations or vice versa, and which molecular defect have a more dominant effect on the clinical behavior of these tumors. It has been suggested that testing for somatic MMR gene mutations should be part of a diagnostic work-up of patients with unresolved abnormal tissue screening results.

In a recent large study of colorectal cancer,[27] mutation-negative patients with MSI-high tumors and loss of MMR proteins by immunohistochemistry (and without *MLH1* promoter hypermethylation) formed a distinct group that, compared with patients with sporadic colorectal cancer, presented at a younger age and showed greater rates of fulfillment of Revised Bethesda Criteria[28] and greater rates of right-sided tumors. In addition, their families had a higher incidence of colorectal and noncolorectal Lynch syndrome tumors. Therefore, it is rational that patients with what has been referred to as Lynch-like syndrome[29,30] should be invited to join cancer prevention surveillance programs available to patients with known deleterious mutations in *MMR* genes.

STRATEGIES AND CHALLENGES OF SCREENING FOR LYNCH SYNDROME IN ENDOMETRIAL CARCINOMA

It is not universally accepted that performing both immunohistochemistry and MSI analysis in tumor screening for Lynch syndrome is necessary. Several different groups have shown that immunohistochemistry alone has a high sensitivity and specificity in identifying endometrial carcinomas with high levels of MSI.[31–35] However, in a recent study of 646 consecutive colorectal (88%), endometrial (7%), and other Lynch syndrome–associated tumors (5%) that underwent MMR immunohistochemistry and MSI testing, it was identified that 12 of 102 (11.8%) MSI-high tumors had intact MMR expression. In contrast, only 1 of 91 (1%) cases with MMR loss was MSS.[10] Based on these results, for optimal detection of all patients with Lynch syndrome, both MSI and immunohistochemistry testing should be performed. As also suggested by others,[36–39] an argument can be made that MSI analysis in colon carcinoma could be used as an initial screen, followed by immunohistochemistry. However, because Lynch syndrome–associated endometrial carcinomas are more often MSI low or MSS, this strategy is not likely to work well for screening patients with endometrial cancer. Therefore, concurrent MSI and MMR immunohistochemistry testing is desirable. If MSI testing is not possible and only MMR immunohistochemistry can be performed, it should be recognized that a small percentage of MSI-high carcinomas will not be captured by performing immunohistochemistry alone.

Although young age at endometrial cancer diagnosis and/or a family history of a Lynch syndrome–related cancer are criteria typically used to pursue further evaluation for Lynch syndrome in patients, it has been shown that, in endometrial cancer, clinical screening tools such as PREMM (Prediction of Mutations in MLH1 and MSH2) (93% sensitivity, 5% specificity), MMRPredict proximal (71% sensitivity, 64% specificity), MMRPredict distal (57% sensitivity, 85% specificity), and MMRPro (57% sensitivity, 85% specificity) miss a significant proportion of patients with Lynch syndrome.[40] This finding is in part caused by some patients with endometrial cancer with Lynch syndrome, and particularly those with *MSH6* mutations, tending not to have first-degree relatives with Lynch syndrome–associated cancers, having endometrial

tumors that are not typically MSI high, and presenting at an older age.[5,12–14,41,42] In addition, as family sizes decrease, the probability of detecting a family history of cancers also decreases. Therefore, universal testing of patients with endometrial cancer will detect Lynch syndrome in a significant proportion of patients who would otherwise have been missed based on age and/or family history.[17]

Early identification of Lynch syndrome in patients with endometrial cancer is essential not only to identify other family members with the syndrome but also in order to proactively manage each patient's own risk of developing subsequent cancers. In particular, for women with Lynch syndrome, endometrial cancer is considered to be a sentinel cancer that precedes colorectal cancer by approximately 1 decade.[43] It is currently recommended that all patients with newly diagnosed colorectal cancer undergo tissue testing for Lynch syndrome regardless of their family or personal history.[44] For endometrial cancer, the Society of Gynecologic Oncology released a clinical practice statement in March of 2014,[45] as follows: "All women who are diagnosed with endometrial cancer should undergo systematic clinical screening for Lynch Syndrome (review of personal and family history) and/or molecular screening. Molecular screening of endometrial cancers for Lynch Syndrome is the preferred strategy when resources are available." A group of European experts (The Mallorca Group) in 2013 recommended testing of all patients with endometrial cancer less than the age of 70 years by immunohistochemistry or MSI analysis.[46]

At the present time, the practice of tumor testing for the purpose of Lynch syndrome identification is highly variable across different centers and countries. Universal tissue testing permits the diagnosis of Lynch syndrome in the highest number of patients compared with other screening strategies and has been implemented in some centers. However, for most others, this entails a significant logistical and financial challenge.[47–49] A study from the United States showed that, although the overall cost of universal testing of patients with endometrial cancer is higher than the overall cost of testing only patients with a 5% to 10% probability of having Lynch syndrome (as defined by Society of Gynecologic Oncology criteria[50]), the cost of testing per every probable Lynch syndrome patient identified is comparable between the two testing strategies. An Australian group has recently proposed a testing approach involving testing of all patients with endometrial carcinoma 60 years of age or younger, as well as testing of older patients with suggestive personal or family history of Lynch syndrome using MSH6 and

PMS2 immunohistochemistry and *MLH1* promoter methylation analysis. This strategy maximizes specificity (93.5%) and sensitivity (100%) of testing, and minimizes cost relative to universal tumor testing using all 4 MMR immunomarkers and *MLH1* methylation analysis.[35] A recent Canadian study corroborated that immunohistochemical testing of all patients younger than 60 years of age yielded high specificity (86.1%) and sensitivity (100%).[34] Screening strategies using immunohistochemistry alone are of particular interest in terms of achieving widespread acceptance, given that MMR immunostains are inexpensive, reliable, accessible, and reproducibly interpretable, whereas MSI and *MLH1* methylation testing is more costly and requires access to a clinical laboratory with expertise in PCR-based analyses.

In addition to the financial challenges of systematic screening of patients with endometrial cancer for Lynch syndrome, success of screening programs also relies on close communication between clinicians, pathologists, geneticists, and patients. For example, in a large cancer center with universal screening for Lynch syndrome through tissue testing, when test results of patients with colorectal cancer were made available to surgeons and genetic counselors, patients who were contacted directly by the genetic counselors on behalf of the treating surgeon had higher rates of referral to genetic testing (100%) compared with those who were not (55%).[51] In addition, beyond the logistical obstacles to systematic tumor screening, several patient factors limit the proportion of patients who decide to proceed with genetic testing after having been identified by tumor tissue testing as having possible Lynch syndrome. These factors include limited health literacy, perceived lack of relevance, being physically and emotionally overwhelmed by diagnosis of cancer, limited insurance coverage (where applicable), and requirement for patient consent.[49,52]

PATHOLOGIC FEATURES OF LYNCH SYNDROME–ASSOCIATED ENDOMETRIAL CANCER

When systematic tissue testing is not possible, tumor tissue testing may be initiated by pathologists or requested by clinicians on a case-by-case basis. In addition to clinical patient information such as patient age of less than 50 years and/or family history of Lynch syndrome–associated tumors, pathologists may use several endometrial tumor features to trigger tumor testing.

Microscopic features in MSI-high colorectal carcinoma have been extensively studied and include poor differentiation, mucinous features, signet ring cell differentiation, mixed tumor histology, tumor cells growing in a medullary-type pattern, increased tumor-infiltrating lymphocyte levels, and a Crohn-like inflammatory infiltrate at the tumor periphery. However, up to 40% of colorectal carcinomas do not have such distinctive microscopic characteristics.[53] The experience with the microscopic features of MSI-high endometrial carcinoma is less than with those of MSI-high colorectal carcinoma.[54–56] In one study, MSI-high endometrial cancers showed higher tumor grade, presence of squamous metaplasia, deeper myometrial invasion, presence of lymphatic/vascular invasion, and extrauterine spread.[55] High numbers of tumor-infiltrating lymphocytes and the presence of peritumoral lymphocytes have been associated with MSI-high status.[54] At the higher numbers of tumor-infiltrating lymphocytes (40 lymphocytes per 10 high-power fields), these counts had a sensitivity of 85% in predicting MSI-high status, but a specificity of only 46%.

Sporadic endometrial carcinomas that are MSI high because of *MLH1* promoter methylation are predominantly endometrioid, especially International Federation of Gynecology and Obstetrics (FIGO) grades 2 and 3, and comprise most (96%) such tumors.[5] However, endometrial carcinomas associated with Lynch syndrome tend to be more histologically diverse and include a much greater proportion of nonendometrioid histotypes, including clear cell, undifferentiated, uterine serous, and mixed carcinoma and carcinosarcoma.[5,56–59] In addition, patients with Lynch syndrome and nonendometrioid tumors tend to be similar in mean age at the time of diagnosis (46.4 years) to those with Lynch syndrome and endometrioid tumors (46.8 years).[5] The patients are considerably younger than the average age of women with nonendometrioid endometrial carcinoma (65–68 years) in the general population.[56,60–64]

Tumor topography may be another clue to the presence of Lynch syndrome. A large series of endometrial carcinomas described a strong association of tumors derived from the lower uterine segment and Lynch syndrome. Thirty-four percent of lower uterine segment tumors were MSI high and 29% had *MMR* gene mutations.[65]

Synchronous carcinomas of the ovary and endometrium tend to occur in younger patients, have lower stage and grade, endometrioid histology, and favorable prognosis.[66–71] Although some investigators have suggested that the presence of such tumor pairs may indicate Lynch syndrome,[56] 2 studies of 45[72] and 59[15] synchronous ovarian and endometrial tumors revealed that only 3.3% to 7% of cases had molecular abnormalities suggestive of Lynch syndrome. Furthermore, in 1 of these studies[15] all tumors identified originated from patients with a prior history or a first-degree relative with a Lynch syndrome–associated cancer. In contrast, in a recent study, 21% of all ovarian non-serous tumors over a 2-year period (with or without concurrent endometrial tumors) in a single institution had MMR immunohistochemical abnormalities. All of the tumors were of endometrioid or clear cell histology.

REFERENCES

1. Kane MF, Loda M, Gaida GM, et al. Methylation of the hMLH1 promoter correlates with lack of expression of hMLH1 in sporadic colon tumors and mismatch repair-defective human tumor cell lines. Cancer Res 1997;57(5):808–11.

2. Herman JG, Umar A, Polyak K, et al. Incidence and functional consequences of hMLH1 promoter hypermethylation in colorectal carcinoma. Proc Natl Acad Sci U S A 1998;95(12):6870–5.

3. Salvesen HB, MacDonald N, Ryan A, et al. Methylation of hMLH1 in a population-based series of endometrial carcinomas. Clin Cancer Res 2000; 6(9):3607–13.

4. Goodfellow PJ, Buttin BM, Herzog TJ, et al. Prevalence of defective DNA mismatch repair and MSH6 mutation in an unselected series of endometrial cancers. Proc Natl Acad Sci U S A 2003;100(10): 5908–13.

5. Broaddus RR, Lynch HT, Chen LM, et al. Pathologic features of endometrial carcinoma associated with HNPCC: a comparison with sporadic endometrial carcinoma. Cancer 2006;106(1):87–94.

6. Boland CR, Fishel R. Lynch syndrome: form, function, proteins, and basketball. Gastroenterology 2005;129(2):751–5.

7. Graham RP, Kerr SE, Butz ML, et al. Heterogenous MSH6 loss is a result of microsatellite instability within MSH6 and occurs in sporadic and hereditary colorectal and endometrial carcinomas. Am J Surg Pathol 2015;39(10):1370–6.

8. Boland CR, Thibodeau SN, Hamilton SR, et al. A National Cancer Institute workshop on microsatellite instability for cancer detection and familial predisposition: development of international criteria for the determination of microsatellite instability in colorectal cancer. Cancer Res 1998;58(22):5248–57.

9. Simpkins SB, Bocker T, Swisher EM, et al. MLH1 promoter methylation and gene silencing is the primary cause of microsatellite instability in sporadic endometrial cancers. Hum Mol Genet 1999;8(4):661–6.

10. Bartley AN, Luthra R, Saraiya DS, et al. Identification of cancer patients with Lynch syndrome: clinically significant discordances and problems in tissue-based mismatch repair testing. Cancer Prev Res (Phila) 2012;5(2):320–7.

11. Kuismanen SA, Moisio AL, Schweizer P, et al. Endometrial and colorectal tumors from patients with hereditary nonpolyposis colon cancer display different patterns of microsatellite instability. Am J Pathol 2002;160(6):1953–8.

12. Berends MJ, Wu Y, Sijmons RH, et al. Molecular and clinical characteristics of MSH6 variants: an analysis of 25 index carriers of a germline variant. Am J Hum Genet 2002;70(1):26–37.

13. Wagner A, Hendriks Y, Meijers-Heijboer EJ, et al. Atypical HNPCC owing to MSH6 germline mutations: analysis of a large Dutch pedigree. J Med Genet 2001;38(5):318–22.

14. Wu Y, Berends MJ, Mensink RG, et al. Association of hereditary nonpolyposis colorectal cancer-related tumors displaying low microsatellite instability with MSH6 germline mutations. Am J Hum Genet 1999; 65(5):1291–8.

15. Soliman PT, Broaddus RR, Schmeler KM, et al. Women with synchronous primary cancers of the endometrium and ovary: do they have Lynch syndrome? J Clin Oncol 2005;23(36):9344–50.

16. Duval A, Hamelin R. Mutations at coding repeat sequences in mismatch repair-deficient human cancers: toward a new concept of target genes for instability. Cancer Res 2002;62(9):2447–54.

17. Bruegl AS, Djordjevic B, Batte B, et al. Evaluation of clinical criteria for the identification of Lynch syndrome among unselected patients with endometrial cancer. Cancer Prev Res (Phila) 2014;7(7):686–97.

18. Leenen CH, van Lier MG, van Doorn HC, et al. Prospective evaluation of molecular screening for Lynch syndrome in patients with endometrial cancer ≤70 years. Gynecol Oncol 2012;125(2):414–20.

19. Backes FJ, Leon ME, Ivanov I, et al. Prospective evaluation of DNA mismatch repair protein expression in primary endometrial cancer. Gynecol Oncol 2009;114(3):486–90.

20. Seiden MV, Patel D, O'Neill MJ, et al. Case records of the Massachusetts General Hospital. Case 13-2007. A 46-year-old woman with gynecologic and intestinal cancers. N Engl J Med 2007; 356(17):1760–9.

21. Ollikainen M, Abdel-Rahman WM, Moisio AL, et al. Molecular analysis of familial endometrial carcinoma: a manifestation of hereditary nonpolyposis colorectal cancer or a separate syndrome? J Clin Oncol 2005;23(21):4609–16.

22. Rhees J, Arnold M, Boland CR. Inversion of exons 1-7 of the MSH2 gene is a frequent cause of unexplained Lynch syndrome in one local population. Fam Cancer 2014;13(2):219–25.

23. Ligtenberg MJ, Kuiper RP, Chan TL, et al. Heritable somatic methylation and inactivation of MSH2 in families with Lynch syndrome due to deletion of the 3' exons of TACSTD1. Nat Genet 2009;41(1): 112–7.

24. Geurts-Giele WR, Leenen CH, Dubbink HJ, et al. Somatic aberrations of mismatch repair genes as a cause of microsatellite-unstable cancers. J Pathol 2014;234(4):548–59.

25. Haraldsdottir S, Hampel H, Tomsic J, et al. Colon and endometrial cancers with mismatch repair deficiency can arise from somatic, rather than germline, mutations. Gastroenterology 2014;147(6):1308–16.e1.

26. Mensenkamp AR, Vogelaar IP, van Zelst-Stams WA, et al. Somatic mutations in MLH1 and MSH2 are a frequent cause of mismatch-repair deficiency in Lynch syndrome-like tumors. Gastroenterology 2014;146(3): 643–6.e8.

27. Rodriguez-Soler M, Perez-Carbonell L, Guarinos C, et al. Risk of cancer in cases of suspected Lynch syndrome without germline mutation. Gastroenterology 2013;144(5):926–32.e1, [quiz: e913–24].

28. Umar A, Boland CR, Terdiman JP, et al. Revised Bethesda Guidelines for hereditary nonpolyposis colorectal cancer (Lynch syndrome) and microsatellite instability. J Natl Cancer Inst 2004;96(4):261–8.

29. Carethers JM. Differentiating Lynch-like from Lynch syndrome. Gastroenterology 2014;146(3):602–4.

30. Boland CR. The mystery of mismatch repair deficiency: Lynch or Lynch-like? Gastroenterology 2013;144(5):868–70.

31. Rosen DG, Cai KQ, Luthra R, et al. Immunohistochemical staining of hMLH1 and hMSH2 reflects microsatellite instability status in ovarian carcinoma. Mod Pathol 2006;19(11):1414–20.

32. Cai KQ, Albarracin C, Rosen D, et al. Microsatellite instability and alteration of the expression of hMLH1 and hMSH2 in ovarian clear cell carcinoma. Hum Pathol 2004;35(5):552–9.

33. Modica I, Soslow RA, Black D, et al. Utility of immunohistochemistry in predicting microsatellite instability in endometrial carcinoma. Am J Surg Pathol 2007;31(5):744–51.

34. Ferguson SE, Aronson M, Pollett A, et al. Performance characteristics of screening strategies for Lynch syndrome in unselected women with newly diagnosed endometrial cancer who have undergone universal germline mutation testing. Cancer 2014; 120(24):3932–9.

35. Buchanan DD, Tan YY, Walsh MD, et al. Tumor mismatch repair immunohistochemistry and DNA MLH1 methylation testing of patients with endometrial cancer diagnosed at age younger than 60 years optimizes triage for population-level germline mismatch repair gene mutation testing. J Clin Oncol 2014;32(2):90–100.

36. Pedroni M, Roncari B, Maffei S, et al. A mononucleotide markers panel to identify hMLH1/hMSH2 germline mutations. Dis Markers 2007;23(3):179–87.

37. Chapusot C, Martin L, Puig PL, et al. What is the best way to assess microsatellite instability status in colorectal cancer? Study on a population base of 462 colorectal cancers. Am J Surg Pathol 2004;28(12): 1553–9.

38. Barrow E, McMahon R, Evans DG, et al. Cost analysis of biomarker testing for mismatch repair deficiency in node-positive colorectal cancer. Br J Surg 2008;95(7):868–75.

39. Arnold CN, Goel A, Compton C, et al. Evaluation of microsatellite instability, hMLH1 expression and hMLH1 promoter hypermethylation in defining the MSI phenotype of colorectal cancer. Cancer Biol Ther 2004;3(1):73–8.

40. Mercado RC, Hampel H, Kastrinos F, et al. Performance of PREMM(1,2,6), MMRpredict, and MMRpro in detecting Lynch syndrome among endometrial cancer cases. Genet Med 2012;14(7):670–80.

41. Hampel H, Frankel W, Panescu J, et al. Screening for Lynch syndrome (hereditary nonpolyposis colorectal cancer) among endometrial cancer patients. Cancer Res 2006;66(15):7810–7.

42. Pineda M, Gonzalez S, Lazaro C, et al. Detection of genetic alterations in hereditary colorectal cancer screening. Mutat Res 2010;693(1–2):19–31.

43. Lu KH, Dinh M, Kohlmann W, et al. Gynecologic cancer as a "sentinel cancer" for women with hereditary nonpolyposis colorectal cancer syndrome. Obstet Gynecol 2005;105(3):569–74.

44. Backes FJ, Hampel H, Backes KA, et al. Are prediction models for Lynch syndrome valid for probands with endometrial cancer? Fam Cancer 2009;8(4): 483–7.

45. SGO. Clinical Practice Statement: Screening for Lynch Syndrome in Endometrial Cancer. 2014. Available at: https://www.sgo.org/clinical-practice/guidelines/screening-for-lynch-syndrome-in-endometrial-cancer/.

46. Vasen HF, Blanco I, Aktan-Collan K, et al. Revised guidelines for the clinical management of Lynch syndrome (HNPCC): recommendations by a group of European experts. Gut 2013;62(6):812–23.

47. Bellcross CA, Bedrosian SR, Daniels E, et al. Implementing screening for Lynch syndrome among patients with newly diagnosed colorectal cancer: summary of a public health/clinical collaborative meeting. Genet Med 2012;14(1):152–62.

48. Kalloger SE, Allo G, Mulligan AM, et al. Use of mismatch repair immunohistochemistry and microsatellite instability testing: exploring Canadian practices. Am J Surg Pathol 2012;36(4):560–9.

49. Beamer LC, Grant ML, Espenschied CR, et al. Reflex immunohistochemistry and microsatellite instability testing of colorectal tumors for Lynch syndrome among US cancer programs and follow-up of abnormal results. J Clin Oncol 2012;30(10):1058–63.

50. Lancaster JM, Powell CB, Kauff ND, et al. Society of Gynecologic Oncologists Education Committee statement on risk assessment for inherited gynecologic cancer predispositions. Gynecol Oncol 2007; 107(2):159–62.

51. Heald B, Plesec T, Liu X, et al. Implementation of universal microsatellite instability and immunohistochemistry screening for diagnosing Lynch syndrome in a large academic medical center. J Clin Oncol 2013;31(10):1336–40.

52. Tomiak E, Samson A, Spector N, et al. Reflex testing for Lynch syndrome: if we build it, will they come? Lessons learned from the uptake of clinical genetics services by individuals with newly diagnosed colorectal cancer (CRC). Fam Cancer 2014;13(1):75–82.

53. Alexander J, Watanabe T, Wu TT, et al. Histopathological identification of colon cancer with microsatellite instability. Am J Pathol 2001;158(2):527–35.

54. Shia J, Black D, Hummer AJ, et al. Routinely assessed morphological features correlate with microsatellite instability status in endometrial cancer. Hum Pathol 2008;39(1):116–25.

55. Honore LH, Hanson J, Andrew SE. Microsatellite instability in endometrioid endometrial carcinoma: correlation with clinically relevant pathologic variables. Int J Gynecol Cancer 2006;16(3):1386–92.

56. Garg K, Shih K, Barakat R, et al. Endometrial carcinomas in women aged 40 years and younger: tumors associated with loss of DNA mismatch repair proteins comprise a distinct clinicopathologic subset. Am J Surg Pathol 2009;33(12):1869–77.

57. Carcangiu ML, Radice P, Casalini P, et al. Lynch syndrome–related endometrial carcinomas show a high frequency of nonendometrioid types and of high FIGO grade endometrioid types. Int J Surg Pathol 2010;18(1):21–6.

58. Djordjevic B, Barkoh BA, Luthra R, et al. Relationship between PTEN, DNA mismatch repair, and tumor histotype in endometrial carcinoma: retained positive expression of PTEN preferentially identifies sporadic non-endometrioid carcinomas. Mod Pathol 2013;26(10):1401–12.

59. Hampel H, Panescu J, Lockman J, et al. Comment on: screening for Lynch syndrome (hereditary nonpolyposis colorectal cancer) among endometrial cancer patients. Cancer Res 2007;67(19):9603.

60. Abeler VM, Kjorstad KE. Clear cell carcinoma of the endometrium: a histopathological and clinical study of 97 cases. Gynecol Oncol 1991;40(3):207–17.

61. Christopherson WM, Alberhasky RC, Connelly PJ. Carcinoma of the endometrium. II. Papillary adenocarcinoma: a clinical pathological study, 46 cases. Am J Clin Pathol 1982;77(5):534–40.

62. Webb GA, Lagios MD. Clear cell carcinoma of the endometrium. Am J Obstet Gynecol 1987;156(6):1486–91.

63. Doss LL, Llorens AS, Henriquez EM. Carcinosarcoma of the uterus: a 40-year experience from the state of Missouri. Gynecol Oncol 1984;18(1):43–53.

64. Olah KS, Dunn JA, Gee H. Leiomyosarcomas have a poorer prognosis than mixed mesodermal tumours when adjusting for known prognostic factors: the result of a retrospective study of 423 cases of uterine sarcoma. Br J Obstet Gynaecol 1992;99(7):590–4.

65. Westin SN, Lacour RA, Urbauer DL, et al. Carcinoma of the lower uterine segment: a newly described association with Lynch syndrome. J Clin Oncol 2008;26(36):5965–71.

66. Zaino R, Whitney C, Brady MF, et al. Simultaneously detected endometrial and ovarian carcinomas–a prospective clinicopathologic study of 74 cases: a gynecologic oncology group study. Gynecol Oncol 2001;83(2):355–62.

67. Eisner RF, Nieberg RK, Berek JS. Synchronous primary neoplasms of the female reproductive tract. Gynecol Oncol 1989;33(3):335–9.

68. Falkenberry SS, Steinhoff MM, Gordinier M, et al. Synchronous endometrioid tumors of the ovary and endometrium. A clinicopathologic study of 22 cases. J Reprod Med 1996;41(10):713–8.

69. Ayhan A, Yalcin OT, Tuncer ZS, et al. Synchronous primary malignancies of the female genital tract. Eur J Obstet Gynecol Reprod Biol 1992;45(1):63–6.

70. Pearl ML, Johnston CM, Frank TS, et al. Synchronous dual primary ovarian and endometrial carcinomas. Int J Gynaecol Obstet 1993;43(3):305–12.

71. Sheu BC, Lin HH, Chen CK, et al. Synchronous primary carcinomas of the endometrium and ovary. Int J Gynaecol Obstet 1995;51(2):141–6.

72. Shannon C, Kirk J, Barnetson R, et al. Incidence of microsatellite instability in synchronous tumors of the ovary and endometrium. Clin Cancer Res 2003;9(4):1387–92.

Testing for Hereditary Predisposition in Patients with Gynecologic Cancers, Quo Vadis?

Gillian Mitchell, MBBS, RCPSC, PhD[a,b,*],
Kasmintan A. Schrader, MBBS, FRCPC, PhD[c,d]

KEYWORDS

• Genetic predisposition • Gynecologic cancer • Multiplex genetic testing • Gene panels

---

Key points

- A clinically important fraction of gynecologic cancers arise due to an inherited predisposition, and more genes predisposing to gynecologic cancers will be discovered in the coming years.

- Advances in technology are increasing access to genetic testing by driving down test costs and enabling the development of gene panel tests.

- Improving access (by improving technology and reducing costs) to somatic genetic tests will be an important route to increase access to germline predisposition testing to more families.

- New models of genetic counseling are necessary if more women with gynecologic cancers and their families are to benefit from cancer predisposition testing.

ABSTRACT

Genetic testing for a hereditary predisposition to gynecologic cancers has been available clinically since the 1990s. Since then, knowledge of the hereditary contribution to gynecologic cancers has dramatically increased, especially with respect to ovarian cancer. Although knowledge of the number of gynecologic cancer–predisposing genes has increased, the integration of genetic predisposition testing into routine clinical practice has been much slower. This article summarizes the technical and practical aspects of genetic testing in gynecologic cancers, the potential barriers to more widespread access and practice of genetic testing for hereditary predisposition to gynecologic cancers, and the potential solutions to these barriers.

OVERVIEW

Genetic testing for a hereditary predisposition to gynecologic cancers has been available as a clinical service since the 1990s with the discovery of the *BRCA1*,[1] *BRCA2*,[2] and mismatch repair genes.[3] Since then, the hereditary contribution to gynecologic cancers has dramatically increased, especially with respect to ovarian cancer.[4,5] Although the number of gynecologic cancer–predisposing genes has increased, the integration of

---

Disclosure Statement: AstraZeneca - Advisory Board member and cochair of industry-sponsored education meeting around BRCA testing in ovarian cancer (G. Mitchell); no disclosures (K.A. Schrader).
[a] Hereditary Cancer Program, BC Cancer Agency, 600 West 10th Ave, Vancouver, British Columbia V5Z 4E6, Canada; [b] Department of Medical Oncology, University of British Columbia, 2329 West Mall, Vancouver, British Columbia V6T 1Z4, Canada; [c] Hereditary Cancer Program, Department of Molecular Oncology, BC Cancer Agency, 600 Wet 10th Ave, Vancouver, British Columbia V5Z 4E6, Canada; [d] Department of Medical Genetics, University of British Columbia, 2329 West Mall, Vancouver, British Columbia V6T 1Z4, Canada
* Corresponding author. Hereditary Cancer Program, BC Cancer Agency, 750 West Broadway, Vancouver, British Columbia V5Z 1H5, Canada.
E-mail address: Gillian.mitchell@bccancer.bc.ca

Surgical Pathology 9 (2016) 301–306
http://dx.doi.org/10.1016/j.path.2016.01.009

genetic predisposition testing into routine clinical practice has been much slower than the pace of discovery of the genes.

This article summarizes the technical and practical aspects of genetic testing in gynecologic cancers, the potential barriers to more widespread access and practice of genetic testing for hereditary predisposition to gynecologic cancers, and the potential solutions to these barriers. Other articles in this issue of *Surgical Pathology Clinics* discuss the specifics of the hereditary contribution to a range of gynecologic cancers.

GENETIC TESTING

The way genetic testing has been undertaken has changed dramatically over the past 20 years. It is important to understand the various historic methods and their sensitivity to finding mutations to appreciate the likelihood of a mutation being missed if a test was performed using one of the older methods and when it is desirable to repeat testing in a family in whom there is a high index of suspicion for a mutation.

Types of pathogenic mutations occurring in cancer predisposition genes include point mutations, which alter only 1 or a few nucleotides along a DNA strand (including deletions, insertions, base changes, and inversions) and these can be nonsense, missense, frameshift, or transcription errors or larger changes to the gene, such as deletions, inversions, and duplications. Nonsense and frameshift mutations commonly give rise to a truncated protein product and/or a protein, which is very different and nonfunctional whereas missense mutations cause an incorrect amino acid to be inserted into the protein, and its effect on protein function depends greatly on which amino acid replaces the native amino acid and the function of that region of the protein. It is often not known whether a missense mutation causes the disease of interest (ie, a pathogenic mutation), and these variants are termed *variants of uncertain significance* (*VUS*).

HISTORIC METHODS

Direct sequence analysis (ie DNA sequencing) is considered the gold standard for mutation testing but historically was limited by its cost and time-consuming nature. Mutation scanning methods initially were used to identify samples likely to harbor a mutation, which could then be sequenced to identify the specific mutation.

The protein truncation test (PTT)[6] is based on many of the pathogenic mutations in cancer predisposition genes resulting in a truncated protein product. The PTT compares the size of products resulting from in vitro transcription and translation of native DNA based on their movement through a gel; if a truncated product is detected, targeted sequencing is then used to investigate the nature of DNA at that point. Heteroduplex analysis (HAD), single-strand conformation polymorphism, and denaturing gradient gel electrophoresis (DGGE) are also scanning methods that exploit the conformational changes in DNA arising from the mutation. Like the PTT, the sensitivity of these techniques is usually less than 75%.[7] Denaturing high-performance liquid chromatography (DHPLC) was a higher throughput technique also based on the formation of heteroduplexes containing the mutation region of DNA, with a higher sensitivity for point mutations reported to be more than 90%, and the reagent costs were approximately 10% to 20% of the cost for sequencing during the early 2000s.[8]

People who had cancer genetic testing years ago using PTT, HAD, DGGE, or DHPLC without a test for large deletions, rearrangement, or duplications and no mutation detected should be offered the opportunity for updated clinical testing using a modern technique with greater sensitivity.

CURRENT TESTING METHODS

With the rapid improvements in technology and resulting reductions in reagent volumes and costs, direct sequencing (Sanger sequencing[9]) became the test of choice for point mutations in most cancer predisposition genes, usually in combination with a test for larger gene deletions and rearrangements (such as multiplex ligation-dependent probe amplification [MLPA][10]), which cannot be detected by Sanger sequencing. The recent advent of massively parallel sequencing (MPS), also known as next-generation sequencing,[11] has enabled a dramatic change in cancer genetic testing, with the ability to test multiple samples for mutations in multiple genes simultaneously (ie in parallel) at much reduced cost and forms the basis of the explosion in availability of cancer gene panel tests. An additional test for large deletions and rearrangements may or may not be necessary when MPS is used; an analysis of copy number change from the MPS readout may be sufficient to diagnose a deletion, rearrangement, or duplication but it is still not universally accepted that copy number change is as reliable as MLPA for these types of mutations. Similarly, there is still debate as to whether a secondary validation test is required to prove the existence of a mutation identified through an MPS-based test, for example, if a Sanger-based confirmation test is needed to confirm the presence of a BRCA mutation found by an MPS-based panel test in a woman with ovarian cancer.

It is, therefore, important for a requesting clinician to understand the methodology used by the testing laboratory and be very familiar with the pros and cons of the technique(s) and whether another test is required to confirm the presence of a mutation.

WHEN IS A GENE READY FOR ROUTINE CANCER PREDISPOSITION TESTING?

Genetic testing for cancer predisposition has been routinely available since the early 1990s since the discovery of the BRCA1[1] and BRCA2[2] genes. The adoption of a gene for routine clinical mutation testing and funding/reimbursement for the test have been cautious because each test has had to fulfill the 3 categories of test performance, namely analytical validity, clinical validity, and clinical utility.[12] Historically, ensuring adherence to these categories before a test is clinically available has been helped by the slow and labor intensive nature of the testing and its high cost, but with the rapid fall in test costs and the ability to test multiple genes at the same time, there is increasing pressure from many sources to start clinical testing for mutations in genes for which there are less robust data in support of their clinical validity and clinical utility. Testing for mutations in genes where the clinical validity and utility are not clearly defined brings with it the risk of misinterpreting the significance of the variant and people undertaking more aggressive cancer risk management than required or not taking appropriate cancer risk management if they are falsely reassured about their cancer risk.

There is no doubt that the slow pace of adoption of genes for routine testing in the past was too slow and many people missed the opportunity to have their cancer predisposition diagnosed, but with the rapid advent of panel testing with the capacity to include multiple genes in every test the pendulum risks swinging too far in the opposite direction, with genes included in panel tests when their clinical utility and validity are not at all clear.[13] It is essential that clinicians ordering genetic tests for their patients understand the nature and strength of the data in support of a gene's proposed role in cancer predisposition to guide their patients appropriately in the event a mutation is found in the gene. Panel tests focused on the more common hereditary cancer predisposition of breast, gynecologic, and bowel cancers are particularly vulnerable to the inclusion of genes for which the data in support of their clinical validity and utility are lacking.

Gathering the data around clinical validity and utility has always been difficult due to the relative rarity of the cancer predisposition genes, making gathering the necessary number of people/families to generate sufficient statistical power to produce robust estimates of risk both time consuming and costly. This has been difficult enough with the more common genes, such as BRCA1 and BRCA2 (predominantly breast and ovarian cancer risk) and the mismatch repair genes MLH1, MSH2, MSH6, and PMS2 (predominantly colorectal, endometrial, and ovarian cancer risks), but is even more problematic with the rarer genes, such as RAD51C and RAD51D (predominantly ovarian cancer risk). The rapidly increasing numbers of people being tested for cancer predisposition, however, and many who are tested using gene panels bring an opportunity to investigate the clinical validity and utility of the more recently discovered and less well-studied genes after the fact, if the appropriate data can be collected linking results and personal and family cancer history and, ideally, with prospective follow-up of people found to have mutations in these genes. One novel initiative in North America, the Prospective Registry of Multiplex Testing (PROMPT) study (https://connect. patientcrossroads.org/?org=prompt), invites people who have had a panel test to sign up and provide details about themselves, their family, and their panel gene results, with the objective of collecting more information about the clinical correlations of mutations in these rarer genes.

SINGLE-GENE VERSUS GENE PANEL VERSUS WHOLE-EXOME VERSUS WHOLE-GENOME APPROACHES TO CLINICAL GENETIC TESTING

There is substantial genetic heterogeneity in the predisposition to many of the common cancers, that is, mutations in a range of genes can result in the same clinical phenotype. For example, nonmucinous ovarian cancer can be associated with mutations in BRCA1, BRCA2, MLH1, MSH2, MSH6, PMS2, TP53, RAD51C, and RAD51D genes and probably PALB2 and BRIP1 as well as a range of other genes in the homologous repair pathway.[4,14] For this reason, single-gene testing for predisposition to the common clinical phenotypes, either testing 1 gene only or testing a series of genes tested 1 after another, is rapidly being superseded by panel testing, where multiple genes can be tested in parallel at a fraction of the cost of testing a series of single genes and in a fraction of the time.[15]

Although the cost and efficiency advantages of panel testing are clear, there are potential drawbacks, or at least issues to address, around panel testing that must be highlighted to patients offered these tests. (1) The inclusion of genes that have yet to have proved clinical validity and utility, as discussed previously. (2) The uncertainty around cancer risk estimates for mutations in a panel gene identified in the absence of the usual clinical phenotype; for example, when a CDH1 pathogenic mutation is identified in a woman with ovarian cancer and no family history of gastric cancer or lobular breast cancer, is the risk of diffuse gastric cancer in her family the same as in other CDH1 carrier families who already have a strong family history of diffuse gastric cancer, and should prophylactic gastrectomy still be offered to her mutation-carrying relatives? (3) The chance of finding gene variants for which the clinical significance is uncertain (VUS); the more genes included in the panel and the inclusion of genes with uncertain clinical validity and utility the more likely that a VUS result is returned. It is essential that VUS are not treated and managed as pathogenic mutations, because a vast majority eventually prove to be benign, and that families are counseled about risk and cancer risk management based on their personal and/or family histories and not on the existence of the VUS.[16]

The use of whole-exome (a test of the coding regions of the majority of genes in the human genome) and whole-genome (a test of coding and noncoding regions of the human genome) approaches to genetic testing for cancer predisposition is rare in routine clinical practice but is occasionally undertaken with informed consent, often in the research setting, when there is a striking clinical phenotype and no mutation identified after more conventional genetic testing approaches.[17,18]

A major issue for both panel tests and the whole-exome/whole-genome approaches is access to good bioinformatics and qualified molecular scientists for the analysis of large volumes of sequence data and their clinical interpretation. Again, clinicians ordering these tests should be aware of the variant calling processes of the laboratory they select to test a patient.

SOMATIC GENETIC TESTING OR GERMLINE GENETIC TESTING?

The majority of cancer predisposition testing is performed on germline material sourced from peripheral blood. Occasionally, germline testing needs to be undertaken on a skin biopsy if a patient has had a bone marrow transplant. With the advent of new therapeutic agents, however, such as poly (ADP-ribose) polymerase (PARP) inhibitors in BRCA-associated cancers, such as ovarian cancer,[19] or programmed cell death protein 1 (PD-1) inhibitors[20] in mismatch repair–deficient tumors (dMMRs), such as endometrial cancer, there is increasing interest in tumor-based genetic testing because these agents seem effective in both the germline and somatically mutated tumors. As government approvals for these targeted agents are delivered, there will be increasing interest in tumor—rather than germline—genetic testing because this will find both types of mutations.[21,22] Furthermore, if there is a therapeutic decision based on the result, this tumour dMMR testing will become more routine, that is, an automatic test without clinician request, at the time of cancer diagnosis just as most colorectal and lung cancers and melanomas are now tested for epidermal growth factor receptors (EGFR), BRAF, and KRAS expression or mutations. The important difference with tumor BRCA or dMMR testing is that identifying somatic BRCA mutations or mismatch repair deficiency brings with it the appreciable likelihood that the detected mutation is a germline mutation, which needs to be managed appropriately; for example, more than 50% of BRCA mutations identified through ovarian tumor testing may prove germline.[23,24] Given the effective risk management strategies available to women with BRCA mutations, it would be unethical not to offer women germline testing if a tumor-based test returned a BRCA mutation; hence, women will need to be appropriately informed about the possibility of detecting a germline mutation and its implications, if reflex tumor testing is to become routine. Novel methods of delivering appropriate levels of information about the test and the ramifications of its result while avoiding overloading a woman newly diagnosed with ovarian cancer and slowing down the processing of patients through the oncology clinics need to be developed because not informing a woman about the potential ramifications ahead of the test is simply not acceptable.

If tumor testing for BRCA mutations is to become routine for therapeutic reasons, by default it will become the primary screen for germline mutations in the ovarian cancer setting, so it is essential that the tumor test has comparable sensitivity for detecting germline mutations as a standard germline test. Concerns about reduced sensitivity for germline mutations has been one of the major concerns around the wider adoption of a tumor-based approach to identifying germline mutation carriers but technical issues are also a barrier, with the quality of DNA varying significantly between tumors depending on the fixation technique and the bioinformatics required to analyze a much more genetically heterogeneous tumor sample compared with a genetically more pure germline sample. Parallel assessment of blood can address these issues.[25] If tumor were the only tissue to be tested consideration would need to be given to the time point of genetic testing to account for potential somatic loss of the germline allele that can be seen.[22]

One important outcome of widespread BRCA tumor testing will be the increasing availability of tumor tests at a more affordable price, which will open up the opportunity for more families to have BRCA testing and take preventive actions if a mutation is found. In many jurisdictions, primarily due to the costs of genetic testing, germline genetic testing in a family is initiated in a person who has had cancer because that is the person most likely to have a mutation if it is present in a family. Hence, it is common to find that genetic testing is not offered to a family if there are no living relatives affected by cancer. This is a particular issue to families with a history of ovarian cancer due to the poor survival from this disease, who are the very families who are most at risk of having a BRCA mutation. Being able to test the ovarian cancer of these deceased relatives will be a major advance for these families and should be more widely available in a few years.

OPTIMIZING ACCESS TO GENETIC TESTING FOR HEREDITARY PREDISPOSITION TO GYNECOLOGIC CANCERS

Germline genetic testing is becoming more acceptable to women with gynecologic cancers, their families, and their treating clinicians, but there are still several barriers limiting access of all eligible women to genetic testing and an important proportion of women are still not accessing genetic testing.[26] These barriers include (1) patient factors, such as lack of knowledge of the benefits of genetic testing, genetic testing not fitting with cultural or spiritual health belief models, and fear of testing; (2) clinician factors, including lack of education, perception of lack of utility for the patient and any benefit being focussed on family members who are not patients of the physician, and a clash with their personal views around genetic testing. The latter are important as; the strength of clinician recommendation is a powerful factor influencing health care decisions and they have the same influence on patients' decisions

around genetic testing[26,27]; (3) systemic barriers are also a factor, with lack of genetic services and the cost of testing and the financing of testing limiting access to those who can afford it or funders (public health or health insurers) restricting access to testing by setting eligibility criteria that may exclude women or families who might still be at risk of having a mutation, such as the previous example in which testing is initiated only in families in some jurisdictions if there is a living relative affected by cancer.

We are starting to overcome these barriers. Public education is improving with greater publicity around the benefits of genetic testing and the normalizing of genetic testing, such as when the actress Angelina Jolie announced that she carried a BRCA mutation and had undertaken risk-reducing surgery.[28,29] Physician awareness of the benefits is also increasing and will be driven further by the wider access to targeted therapies, such as PARP inhibitors and PD-1 inhibitors. New models of genetic counseling and testing are being trialed to streamline the process and service more patients,[30,31] and an important first steps will be to offer more widespread index genetic testing to unaffected family members of deceased ovarian cancer patients and testing of tumor specimens of deceased patients. One of the most important solutions, however, is the continuing dropping of the cost of genetic testing (germline-based or tumor-based) without which the increasing numbers of people requesting testing will not be served.

In conclusion, gynecologic cancers have a high heritable fraction and many of the inherited cancer syndromes associated with gynecologic cancers have effective cancer risk management strategies available and new targeted chemotherapeutics will be approved in the coming years. This all means that every patient with gynecologic cancers should be assessed for an inherited cancer predisposition and that genetic testing should be available to all patients determined at risk of a cancer predisposition syndrome and, in turn, their family members if a mutation is identified. Advances in technology are driving down test costs and expanding access to testing through gene panels and tumor-based testing, but more still needs to be done to ensure access to these tests and that the quality of the tests and their interpretation is maintained.

REFERENCES

1. Miki Y, Swensen J, Shattuck-Eidens D, et al. A strong candidate for the breast and ovarian cancer susceptibility gene BRCA1. Science 1994;266(5182):66–71.

2. Wooster R, Neuhausen S, Mangion J, et al. Localisation of a breast cancer susceptibility gene (BRCA2) to chromosome 13q by genetic linkage analysis. Science 1994;265:2088–90.

3. Lynch HT, Snyder CL, Shaw TG, et al. Milestones of Lynch syndrome: 1895-2015. Nat Rev Cancer 2015; 15(3):181–94.

4. Kanchi KL, Johnson KJ, Lu C, et al. Integrated analysis of germline and somatic variants in ovarian cancer. Nat Commun 2014;5:3156.

5. Walsh CS. Two decades beyond BRCA1/2: Homologous recombination, hereditary cancer risk and a target for ovarian cancer therapy. Gynecol Oncol 2015;137(2):343–50.

6. Hauss O, Muller O. The protein truncation test in mutation detection and molecular diagnosis. Methods Mol Biol 2007;375:151–64.

7. Cotton RG. Current methods of mutation detection. Mutat Res 1993;285(1):125–44.

8. Takashima H, Boerkoel CF, Lupski JR. Screening for mutations in a genetically heterogeneous disorder: DHPLC versus DNA sequence for mutation detection in multiple genes causing Charcot-Marie-Tooth neuropathy. Genet Med 2001;3(5):335–42.

9. Sanger F, Nicklen S, Coulson AR. DNA sequencing with chain-terminating inhibitors. Proc Natl Acad Sci U S A 1977;74(12):5463–7.

10. Bunyan DJ, Eccles DM, Sillibourne J, et al. Dosage analysis of cancer predisposition genes by multiplex ligation-dependent probe amplification. Br J Cancer 2004;91(6):1155–9.

11. Tucker T, Marra M, Friedman JM. Massively parallel sequencing: the next big thing in genetic medicine. Am J Hum Genet 2009;85(2):142–54.

12. Burke W. Genetic tests: clinical validity and clinical utility. Curr Protoc Hum Genet 2014;81:9.15.1–9.15.8.

13. Easton DF, Pharoah PD, Antoniou AC, et al. Gene-panel sequencing and the prediction of breast-cancer risk. N Engl J Med 2015;372(23):2243–57.

14. Walsh T, Casadei S, Lee MK, et al. Mutations in 12 genes for inherited ovarian, fallopian tube, and peritoneal carcinoma identified by massively parallel sequencing. Proc Natl Acad Sci U S A 2011; 108(44):18032–7.

15. Kurian AW, Hare EE, Mills MA, et al. Clinical evaluation of a multiple-gene sequencing panel for hereditary cancer risk assessment. J Clin Oncol 2014; 32(19):2001–9.

16. Eccles DM, Mitchell G, Monteiro AN, et al. BRCA1 and BRCA2 genetic testing-pitfalls and recommendations for managing variants of uncertain clinical significance. Ann Oncol 2015;26(10): 2057–65.

17. Schrader KA, Stratton KL, Murali R, et al. Genome sequencing of multiple primary tumors reveals a novel PALB2 variant. J Clin Oncol 2016;34(8):e61–7.

18. Scollon S, Bergstrom K, Kerstein RA, et al. Obtaining informed consent for clinical tumor and germline exome sequencing of newly diagnosed childhood cancer patients. Genome Med 2014;6(9):69.

19. Ledermann J, Harter P, Gourley C, et al. Olaparib maintenance therapy in patients with platinum-sensitive relapsed serous ovarian cancer: a pre-planned retrospective analysis of outcomes by BRCA status in a randomised phase 2 trial. Lancet Oncol 2014;15(8):852–61.

20. Le DT, Uram JN, Wang H, et al. PD-1 blockade in tumors with mismatch-repair deficiency. N Engl J Med 2015;372(26):2509–20.

21. Hyman DH, Solit DB, Arcila ME, et al. Precision medicine at Memorial Sloan Kettering Cancer Center: clinical next-generation sequencing enabling next-generation targeted therapy trials. Drug Discov Today 2015;20(12):1422–8.

22. Schrader KA, Cheng DT, Joseph V, et al. Germline variants in targeted tumor sequencing using matched normal DNA. JAMA Oncol 2016;2(1):104–11.

23. Geisler JP, Hatterman-Zogg MA, Rathe JA, et al. Frequency of BRCA1 dysfunction in ovarian cancer. J Natl Cancer Inst 2002;94(1):61–7.

24. Hilton JL, Geisler JP, Rathe JA, et al. Inactivation of BRCA1 and BRCA2 in ovarian cancer. J Natl Cancer Inst 2002;94(18):1396–406.

25. Jones S, Anagnostou V, Lytle K, et al. Personalized genomic analyses for cancer mutation discovery and interpretation. Sci Transl Med 2015;7(283):283ra53.

26. Armstrong J, Toscano M, Kotchko N, et al. Utilization and outcomes of BRCA genetic testing and counseling in a national commercially insured population: The ABOUT Study. JAMA Oncol 2015;1(9):1251–60.

27. Schwartz MD, Lerman C, Brogan B, et al. Utilization of BRCA1/BRCA2 mutation testing in newly diagnosed breast cancer patients. Cancer Epidemiol Biomarkers Prev 2005;14(4):1003–7.

28. James PA, Mitchell G, Bogwitz M, et al. The Angelina Jolie effect. Med J Aust 2013;199(10):646.

29. Evans DG, Barwell J, Eccles DM, et al. The Angelina Jolie effect: how high celebrity profile can have a major impact on provision of cancer related services. Breast Cancer Res 2014;16(5):442.

30. Slade I, Riddell D, Turnbull C, et al, MCG Programme. Development of cancer genetic services in the UK: A national consultation. Genome Med 2015;7(1):18.

31. Rahman N. Mainstreaming genetic testing of cancer predisposition genes. Clin Med 2014;14(4):436–9.

Prophylactic Gynecologic Specimens from Hereditary Cancer Carriers

Patricia A. Shaw, MD, FRCP(C)[a,b,*],
Blaise A. Clarke, MBBCh, MSc, FRCP(C)[a,b]

KEYWORDS

- Risk-reducing salpingectomy • Salpingo-oophorectomy • BRCA • Lynch syndrome
- Prophylactic surgery • Hereditary cancer • Endometrial cancer • Ovarian cancer

Key points

- Risk-reducing surgery, including salpingo-oophorectomy and hysterectomy, is becoming increasingly common as more women are identified as being at genetic risk for endometrial and/or tubal/ovarian cancer.
- The distal end of the fallopian tube and the fimbria from all salpingectomy specimens should be processed to maximize histologic assessment of tubal epithelium.
- The recognition and classification of high-grade serous carcinoma precursor lesions in the tube are more accurate with the addition of immunohistochemistry.

ABSTRACT

Hereditary breast ovarian cancer and Lynch/hereditary nonpolyposis colorectal cancer syndrome account for most hereditary gynecologic cancers. In the absence of effective cancer screening and other preventative strategies, risk-reducing surgery in women who are known to be at genetic risk of BRCA-associated or of Lynch syndrome carcinomas is effective in significantly decreasing the lifetime risk of developing malignancy. Reflex genomic testing of high-grade ovarian cancers and reflex immunohistochemistry in endometrial cancers will lead to greater recognition of germline-associated cancers. Approaches to processing surgical specimens, the recognition and classification of cancer precursor lesions, and differentiation from their mimics are discussed.

OVERVIEW

Hereditary gynecologic cancers are largely accounted for by 2 syndromes: hereditary breast ovarian cancer (HBOC), and Lynch/hereditary nonpolyposis colorectal cancer syndrome. As with other hereditary syndromes, it is now apparent that the traditional clinical features of multiple affected family members, multiple types of cancers, and early age of onset underestimate the incidence of cancers associated with inherited mutations. A recent study indicated that 24% of unselected ovarian cancers were associated with germline mutations, and that more than 30% of these mutation carriers had no known family history.[1]

Mutations of *BRCA1* and *BRCA2* account for most ovarian, tubal, and peritoneal cancers in HBOC. Inherited mutations of the BRCA genes

Disclosure Statement: The authors have nothing to disclose.
[a] Department of Laboratory Medicine and Pathobiology, University of Toronto, Toronto, Ontario, Canada;
[b] Department of Pathology, University Health Network, Toronto, Ontario, Canada
* Corresponding author. Department of Pathology, University Health Network, Eaton wing, room 11-444, 200 Elizabeth St, Toronto, Ontario M5G 2C4, Canada.
E-mail address: Patricia.shaw@uhn.ca

increase the lifetime risk of developing ovarian/tubal/peritoneal carcinoma from 1.39% in the general population to 40% to 60% (BRCA1) and 11% to 27% (BRCA2) in mutation carriers. High-grade serous carcinoma (HGSC) is the histotype most consistently associated with BRCA1 and BRCA2 mutations, and as many as 25% of women with a diagnosis of HGSC carry a germline mutation.[1–3] Other rare germline mutations have been reported in HGSC with some familial risk, most of which encode proteins that have roles in BRCA1/BRCA2 DNA repair pathways, including BARD1, BRIP1, RAD50, RAD51C, RAD51D, and PALB2.[1,4] A significant percentage of familial ovarian cancers are not associated with known deleterious mutations, and it is likely that other less common and less penetrant genetic risk factors have not yet been discovered.

Screening for HGSC has been shown to be ineffective in reducing mortality, and although the use of oral contraception has been demonstrated to reduce risk in both sporadic and BRCA-associated ovarian cancers, risk-reducing salpingo-oophorectomy (RRSO) is the most effective preventative method. Risk-reducing surgery decreases the risk of HGSC by 90%, but also reduces cancer-related mortality and overall mortality.[5] The term "risk-reducing salpingo-oophorectomy" is favored over prophylactic oophorectomy, reflecting (i) the inclusion of fallopian tube carcinoma in the BRCA-mutation associated cancer phenotype and (ii) the fact that a small percentage of women undergoing preventative surgery continues to have a small risk of developing carcinoma despite removal of the ovaries and fallopian tubes.[6] Carcinomas of the uterus do not appear to be associated with this syndrome, and therefore, prophylactic hysterectomy is not routinely performed in these women.

Current guidelines from the National Comprehensive Cancer Network and the Society of Gynecologic Oncologists advise that RRSO take place between the ages 35 and 40. However, most women known to be at risk do not undergo surgical intervention before the recommended age, in part due to variations in assessment of risk, availability of genetic counseling and testing, and concerns related to early surgical menopause. In addition, only a small percentage of carriers are identified, and despite current recommendations to refer women with epithelial ovarian cancer for genetic counseling and elective genetic testing,[7] only a minority of women with a new diagnosis of high-grade serous carcinoma is tested in most jurisdictions, and therefore, many women at genetic risk are not currently identified.

Lynch syndrome (LS), the most common hereditary cancer syndrome, is an autosomal-dominant disorder associated with germline mutations in DNA mismatch repair genes. The most frequently affected genes are hMLH1, hMSH2, hMSH6, and, less commonly, hPMS2, and mutations in these genes usually lead to microsatellite instability. Microsatellite instability is frequent in endometrial cancer, about 20% to 25%, but in most cases, this is due to hMLH1 promoter hypermethylation and is not reflective of an inherited disorder.

Women with LS have a 60% lifetime risk of endometrial carcinoma, and a 12% risk of ovarian cancer, and in women, the diagnosis of the gynecologic cancer may be the sentinel event indicating the association with LS.[8] Although affected women are at increased lifetime risk for ovarian cancer, the proportion of ovarian cancers associated with LS is relatively low.[1]

Reflex screening of appropriate cancer samples (namely colon and endometrial cancers) with mismatch repair immunohistochemistry to triage patients for LS testing is rapidly becoming standard of care.[9–11] Furthermore, subtype-specific reflex testing strategies have been proposed for ovarian cancer, with some centers performing reflex testing on endometrioid, clear cell, and undifferentiated ovarian carcinomas.[12] LS has implications for both the patient and family members. Because a gynecologic cancer will be the sentinel malignancy in about 60% of women with LS, identification will allow enrollment of these patients in high-risk colon cancer screening programs, which are highly effective.[8] Mismatch repair deficiency, whether of sporadic or hereditary cause, can also inform therapeutic options, such as the use of immune checkpoint inhibitors.[13] Cascade testing of family members to identify unaffected carriers is also critical to facilitate cancer screening and prophylactic surgery in relatives.[14] An added imperative is the potential cost savings for the health care system. As such, with the advent of reflex testing and the drive to identify unaffected family members, prophylactic gynecologic specimens from LS carriers are likely to become more common.

There are other less common and less well-known syndromes associated with gynecologic tumor risk. Cowden syndrome, associated with germline mutations of PTEN, increases the lifetime risk of endometrial carcinoma to19% to 28% by age 70.[15] Mutations in STK11/LKB1 are associated with Peutz-Jeghers syndrome, with an increased risk of adenoma malignum of the cervix and of sex cord stromal tumors of the ovary. Li-Fraumeni syndrome, with germline mutations of

TP53, was not previously thought to be associated with ovarian or uterine malignancies, but a recent publication discovered germline mutations of TP53 in a small percentage of tubal carcinomas. Germline mutations in the *DICER1* and *SMARCA4* genes have been identified to be associated with Sertoli-Leydig tumors and ovarian small cell carcinoma.

Currently, genetic testing in North America for gynecologic cancer risk is restricted, with referral for testing and counseling based on family history and/or histotype of cancer in a first-degree relative. Criteria for genetic testing vary according to jurisdiction. Testing is currently focused on expensive gene-by-gene testing and does not necessarily capture most women either at risk or with a diagnosis of carcinoma that may be associated with an inherited mutation. The combination of reflex immunohistochemistry for MMR proteins in new diagnoses of endometrial carcinoma, and the increasing availability of less expensive and more comprehensive multi-gene panel testing, will increase the identification of families with germline cancer-predisposition genes. In the absence of effective screening techniques for many of the cancers associated with the hereditary syndromes, prophylactic surgeries will increase and will not be restricted to academic centers.

MUTATIONS OF *BRCA1* AND *BRCA2* AND PREVENTION OF HIGH-GRADE SEROUS CARCINOMA

Histopathological review of RRSO specimens in BRCA1/2 mutation carriers has changed the paradigm of HGSC cause and pathogenesis. The detection of occult carcinomas in the fallopian tube led to more comprehensive histopathological assessment of tubal epithelium and subsequently to the identification and classification of serous cancer precursors in the distal fallopian tube and fimbria, which in turn has led to the recognition that the origin of most cases of HGSC is tubal epithelium, not the ovarian surface epithelium.[16–22] The understanding of the pathobiology of the events preceding clinically evident HGSC continues to evolve.

The standard for preventative surgery in BRCA1/2 mutation carriers and for women with an increased risk based on family history is bilateral salpingo-oophorectomy, which includes removal of the tube to the uterine cornua. Some women also undergo hysterectomy, which does not add additional protection against developing BRCA-associated cancers. The concept of a tubal origin of HGSC has recently led to proposals that HGSC risk in mutation carriers may be reduced through bilateral salpingectomy with ovarian retention (BSOR), a procedure that removes the fallopian tubes, including the high anatomic risk portion, the fimbriae, but leaves the ovarian tissue in situ. It is a strategy that would avoid the deleterious health effects of premenopausal oophorectomy and may be viewed as a temporary risk-reducing strategy in younger women, who would be able to complete the risk-reducing surgery at a later age. However, there is as of yet no concrete evidence that this approach in high-risk women is an effective risk-reducing approach, and BSOR is for now considered by many to be investigational. Nevertheless, it is a procedure that may be offered to premenopausal women refusing RRSO.

A third preventative and yet unproved strategy is being used for women with no known genetic risk. Opportunistic salpingectomy has been recommended for all women undergoing tubal ligation or hysterectomy, or other pelvic surgery.[7] Until BSOR has been studied with long-term outcomes in BRCA mutation carriers, opportunistic salpingectomy should be restricted to women at no known genetic risk.[23,24]

Salpingo-oophorectomy specimens for prevention of BRCA-associated tubal/ovarian/peritoneal carcinoma may include

1. RRSO in women at known increased genetic risk of carcinoma (includes pelvic washings)
2. Salpingectomy with ovarian retention (SOR) in women at known increased genetic risk of carcinoma, (includes pelvic washings)
3. Opportunistic salpingectomy in women at no known familial/genetic risk of carcinoma, but undergoing pelvic surgery for other reasons

PROCESSING OF RISK-REDUCING SALPINGO-OOPHORECTOMY SPECIMENS

RRSO will be increasingly adopted as a preventative strategy in women at high genetic risk and is performed in both academic and community practice settings. Because there is a significant incidence of occult carcinoma in RRSO and SOR specimens, the pathologist plays a key role in the multidisciplinary care of women undergoing prophylactic surgery. It is therefore important that pathologists standardize the processing of resected tubal specimens and that the reason for surgery be communicated to the pathologist so the RRSO/SOR specimens are handled and processed to preserve and maximize histologic assessment of the tubal and the ovarian surface epithelium.

To this end, Crum and colleagues outlined a protocol for sectioning and extensively examining the fimbriated end of the fallopian tube (SEE-FIM), devised to optimize the surface area of the high-risk tubal epithelium for microscopic examination.[19] To ensure optimal fixation times for interpretation of subsequent immunohistochemistry, all salpingectomy specimens are fixed for 24 to 48 hours. In 2007, the Association of Directors of Anatomic and Surgical Pathology recommended a 2-tier approach to examination of the fallopian tube, depending on the level of suspicion for an occult invasive or intraepithelial carcinoma.[25] However, because there is a risk of serous tubal intraepithelial carcinoma (STIC), albeit low, and occult carcinoma in women considered to be at low genetic risk of HGSC, it has been recommended that any resected tubal fimbriae be examined following an SEE-FIM-like protocol, and this is the authors' current practice.[22,26]

1. All salpingectomy specimens, including those not known to be associated with a risk of carcinoma:
   a. Fix for a minimum of 24 to 48 hours with care in the handling of the fimbriated ends, protecting the integrity of the fimbrial epithelium.
   b. The distal 2 cm of the fimbriated end is transected.
   c. The fimbria is serially sectioned longitudinally parallel to the long axis, at 2-mm intervals.
   d. The fimbriated end is submitted in toto for histologic examination. Block number of the fimbria is noted.
   e. Histology
      i. A single hematoxylin and eosin (H&E) is taken from each block.
2. RRSO/salpingectomy with ovarian retention: As above plus:
   a. The remainder of the tube is sectioned at 2-mm (maximum) cross-sections.
   b. All sections of the fallopian tube are submitted in toto.
   c. Histology
      i. Infundibulum/fimbria blocks:
         1 H&E plus p53 plus Ki67
         or
         1 H&E plus unstained sections
      ii. A single H&E is taken from each of the remaining blocks.

It is the authors' practice for all RRSO specimens to prepare 1 H&E section plus p53 and Ki67 sections in infundibulum/fimbria blocks. It has been their experience that detection of small STIC lesions may be missed on H&E examination alone, but with the addition of p53 and Ki67 immunohistochemistry a small precursor lesion will be detected. An alternative is to include unstained sections from the same ribbon strip as the H&E section. Assessment of microscopic suspicious lesions may be compromised if additional sections are not included in the initial sectioning of the tissue blocks. Finally, in most circumstances, multistep deeper level sectioning is not necessary, but may be performed if peritoneal washings are positive for malignant cells, and no lesion is detected in initial tube/ovary sections.[27]

GROSS FEATURES

Most patients undergoing prophylactic salpingo-oophorectomy will have been assessed clinically for the presence of malignancy, by transvaginal pelvic ultrasound and possibly by serum CA125, so that in most cases there are no significant macroscopic abnormalities in the resected tubes and ovaries. Occult cancers may rarely be detected on careful macroscopic examination, and the clinically undetected tumor nodules usually involve the tubal fimbria, distal fallopian tube, or ovarian surface. Note should be made of the presence or absence of tubal fimbria (Fig. 1).

OCCULT HIGH-GRADE SEROUS CARCINOMA

By definition, occult carcinoma is not detected preoperatively, and transvaginal ultrasound and serum CA125 are frequently reported as normal within the year prior to RRSO. The first reports of occult carcinoma in BRCA mutation carriers indicated a range of 2.3% to 10.4% incidence of occult carcinoma at the time of RRSO, and there was a surprisingly high incidence of carcinomas involving the distal end, fimbria, of the fallopian tubes.[18,28–30] The frequency is higher in reports when examination of the fallopian tubes and ovaries are performed by meticulous fine sectioning and by consistent review limited to gynecologic pathologists at a single institution, and lower in multi-institution studies without centralized pathology review. The incidence also varies with age of the patient at the time of RRSO and is more frequent with documented germline mutations of BRCA1/2, more frequent with *BRCA1* than *BRCA2* mutations, type of mutation (known deleterious), and according to some studies, whether the patient has a prior history of breast cancer.[31,32]

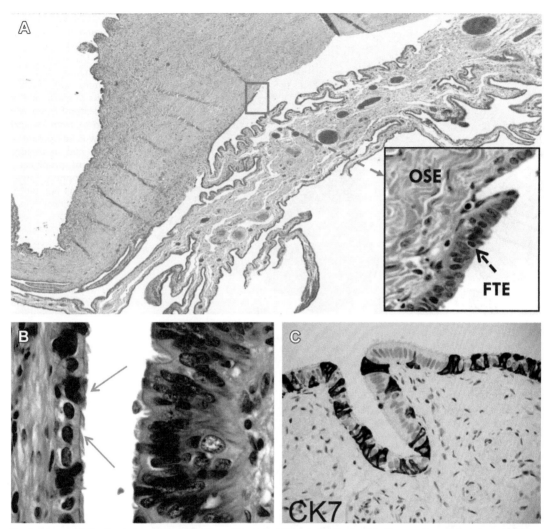

Fig. 1. Normal fallopian tube. (*A*) Single plica of the tubal fimbria is attached to the ovarian surface. Insert shows a higher magnification with a transition from tubal-type epithelium (FTE) to ovarian surface epithelium (OSE). (*B*) Normal tubal mucosa with varied stratification and a mixture of ciliated and secretory cells (*arrows*). (*C*) CK7 immunohistochemistry highlights the distribution of secretory cells (CK7 positive) and ciliated cells (CK7 negative).

MICROSCOPIC

Occult carcinomas in RRSO specimens are usually classified as HGSC.[18,32,33] Like clinically evident HGSC, morphologic features vary and the tumor architecture may include any combination of solid, papillary, or glandular patterns. Nuclear atypia is high grade, often with marked pleomorphism. Mitotic activity may be high, but the size of tumor generally precludes a formal mitotic count.

Immunohistochemistry is useful in confirming histotype. Most tumors have strong nuclear positivity for PAX8 and WT1 and have an abnormal pattern of p53 (diffuse nuclear overexpression or null pattern of expression) reflective of the presence of a mutation in the tumor suppressor gene *TP53*. In addition, the occult carcinomas may show diffuse intense staining for p16, reflecting abrogation of the RB pathway and variable positivity for estrogen receptor.

Even though these tumors are not detected clinically, the stage of the carcinoma when diagnosed ranges from stage 1A to 3C.[29,33–35] Because many of the carcinomas involve the distal end of the fallopian tube, there may also be deposits of tumor on the ovarian surface (**Fig. 2**).[18] Although many of the occult carcinomas are small, and total volume of disease is low, these tumors have a significant risk of recurrence, reported to be as high as 43%.[35,36]

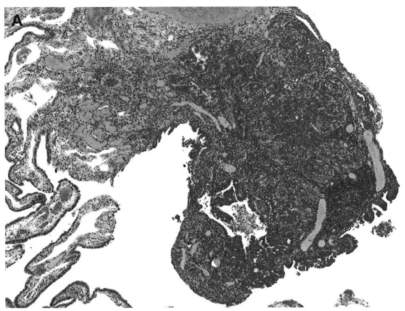

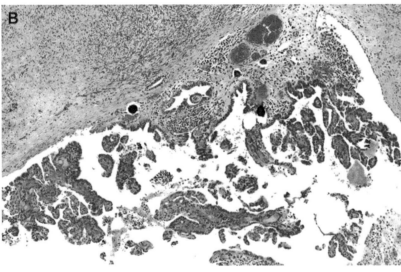

Fig. 2. Occult invasive carcinoma in a 44-year-old BRCA1 mutation carrier. (*A*) HGSC in the tubal fimbria, measuring 1.6 mm. (*B*) Surface deposits of carcinoma on the ipsilateral ovary. (*Reprinted from* Finch A, Shaw P, Rosen B, et al. Clinical and pathologic findings of prophylactic salpingo-oophorectomies in 159 BRCA1 and BRCA2 carriers. Gynecol Oncol 2006;100(1):62; with permission.)

SEROUS TUBAL INTRAEPITHELIAL CARCINOMA

STIC is defined as a localized lesion characterized by morphologic atypia, abnormal p53 expression (reflecting the presence of a p53 mutation), and increased proliferation rate.[37,38] Intraepithelial carcinomas of the tube had been well recognized for many years,[39] but Piek and colleagues[16] made the first convincing description of histologic abnormalities in tubal epithelium of BRCA mutation carriers, in the absence of associated HGSC, supporting the currently favored theory that STIC is the

immediate precursor of HGSC. Several terms have been used to describe atypical tubal lesions in the past, including dysplasia, atypical mucosal epithelial proliferation, and carcinoma in situ.[16,39,40] STIC designates a noninvasive intraepithelial lesion, which resembles HGSC, sharing both morphologic and many molecular features, including the presence of a p53 mutation, an abnormality that has high concordance with abnormal protein expression by immunohistochemistry, a useful feature in the classification of tubal precancerous lesions. The pattern of p53 expression by immunohistochemistry is highly concordant with the type of p53 mutation present.[41] Diffuse intense staining in STIC corresponds with missense mutations (over-accumulation of abnormal protein) and complete loss of staining corresponds to null mutations (due to splice, frameshift, and nonsense muta-tions). Weak, patchy, or isolated cell positivity cor-responds to wild-type *TP53*. Complete loss of staining may be identified in contrast to wild-type focal weak positivity in the background uninvolved tubal epithelium.

STIC may be detected in any 1 of the 3 following clinical settings:

i. In prophylactic salpingectomy specimens from BRCA1/2 mutation carriers
ii. Associated with HGSC of presumed ovarian, tubal, peritoneal origins, reported in up to 60% cases[42–44]
iii. Rarely as an incidental finding in routine surgi-cal specimens[22,26]

MICROSCOPIC

Many STIC lesions are small, making the recogni-tion and accurate diagnostic classification some-times challenging. Like HGSC, STIC has variable histologic features, and the morphologic spectrum of changes is broad. STIC lesions have varying degrees of stratification, and some STIC have exfoliation of cells, sometimes with a growth pattern reminiscent of the slitlike spaces, epithelial "fractures" seen so commonly in the invasive counterpart (Fig. 3A). Detachment of malignant-appearing cells may be associated with superficial implants of the ipsilateral ovary (Fig. 3B).

The reproducibility of the diagnosis using morphologic criteria alone is only moderate among experienced gynecologic pathologists.[45,46] Using current definitions, which include the use of immu-nohistochemistry to improve diagnostic reproduc-ibility, all cases of STIC have the following:

1. Morphologic atypia, which includes not neces-sarily all but a combination of the following features: nuclear enlargement, hyperchroma-sia, irregularly distributed chromatin, nucleolar prominence, loss of polarity, apoptosis, epithe-lial tufting, and mitotic activity
2. Abnormal p53 expression by immunohistochemistry
3. Increased proliferation, with at least 10% of lesion nuclei expressing Ki67 by immunohisto-chemistry (Figs. 4–6).

A diagnostic algorithm using both morphologic features and immunohistochemistry for 2 bio-markers has been shown to improve the reproducibility of the diagnosis of tubal precursor lesions, independent of the pathologist's level of experience (Fig. 7).[38,46] In brief, suspected tubal precursor lesions are first assessed by morpho-logic criteria and categorized as the following:

i. Not suspicious for STIC
ii. Suspicious for STIC
iii. Unequivocal for STIC.

Immunostains for p53 and Ki67 are used to further categorize the lesion:

A diagnosis of STIC requires that a lesion is assessed:

i. To be suspicious for STIC or unequivocal for STIC
   and
ii. To have an abnormal p53 staining pattern, either intense nuclear positivity in greater than 75% of the lesional cells or 0% labeling (null pattern)
    and
iii. To have increased proliferation as indicated by greater than 10% of the lesional cells showing positive Ki67 staining

Lesions not meeting all of these criteria are not diagnosed as STIC, but, following the algo-rithm, would be classified as serous tubal intraepi-thelial lesion (STIL), or p53 signature, or normal/reactive.

Although STIC is a noninvasive lesion, the cells in some cases have the propensity for metastasis without the requirement of invasion into adjacent stroma before peritoneal spread. The morphologic features of STIC and the molecular associations reported to date suggest that STIC is a malignant lesion, and some have recommended that STIC be staged as serous carcinoma, stage 1A.[47] The clinical outcome of patients with STIC, in the absence of positive peritoneal washings or other disease, is not yet well understood and cannot be accurately predicted for an individual patient. There is at least one published report of a patient with an STIC but no evidence of invasive disease recurring with advanced stage disease.[36] One small series indicates a favorable outcome.[48] Nevertheless, although current information does not yet provide clear direction on how patients with an STIC diagnosis should be managed, the accurate diagnosis of STIC clearly has significant clinical implications. Because STICs share molec-ular and genetic alterations with HGSC, and at least 15% of HGSC are associated with germline mutations of *BRCA1* or *BRCA2*, patients with an incidental diagnosis of STIC may also have a higher risk of carrying a germline mutation, and

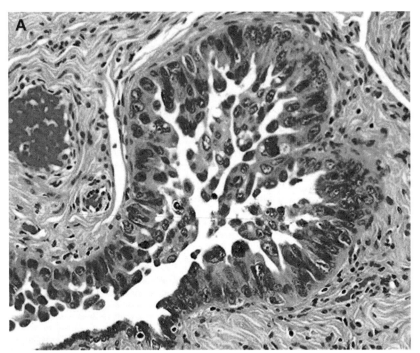

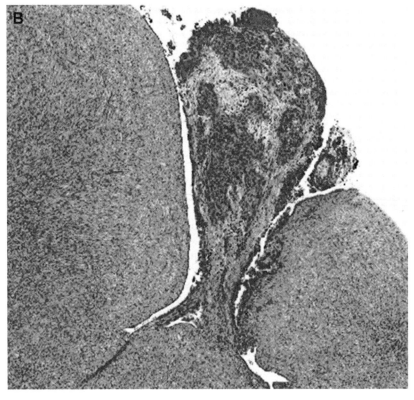

Fig. 3. Serous tubal intra-epithelial lesion (STIC). (*A*) This lesion has prominent tufting, with cell detachment. (*B*) A microscopic focus of HGSC on the ipsilateral ovarian surface. (*From* Shaw PA, Clarke B, George S. Precursor lesions of high grade serous carcinoma. In: Fadare O, editor. Precancerous lesions of the gynecologic tract: diagnostic and molecular genetic pathology. Switzerland: Springer International Publishing, 2016; with permission.)

therefore, referral to a genetic counselor is indicated. Some patients may be offered adjuvant treatment including chemotherapy, so it is important to not overcall this diagnosis.

There is considerable variation in the reported incidence of STIC in RRSO specimens. This variation is due to several factors, particularly study design. Study populations vary widely; some are

Fig. 4. Serous tubal intraepithelial carcinoma (STIC). (*A*) This lesion is recognizable as abnormal at low power magnification (*arrow*). (*B*) Immunohistochemistry for p53 shows diffuse nuclear overexpression. (*C*) Immunohistochemistry for Ki67 shows increased expression, present in greater than 10% of lesion cells.

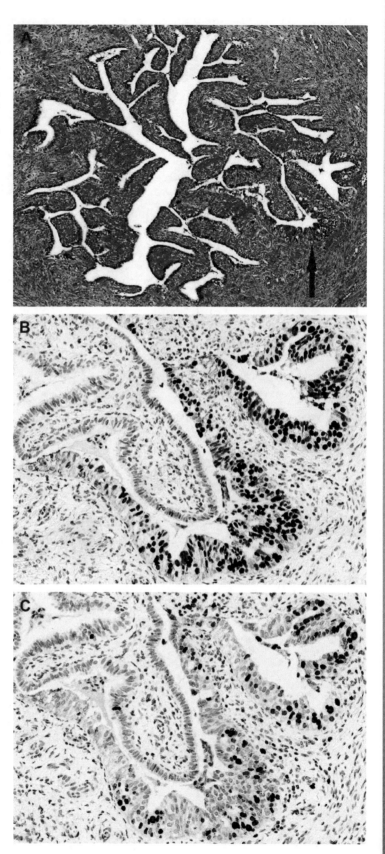

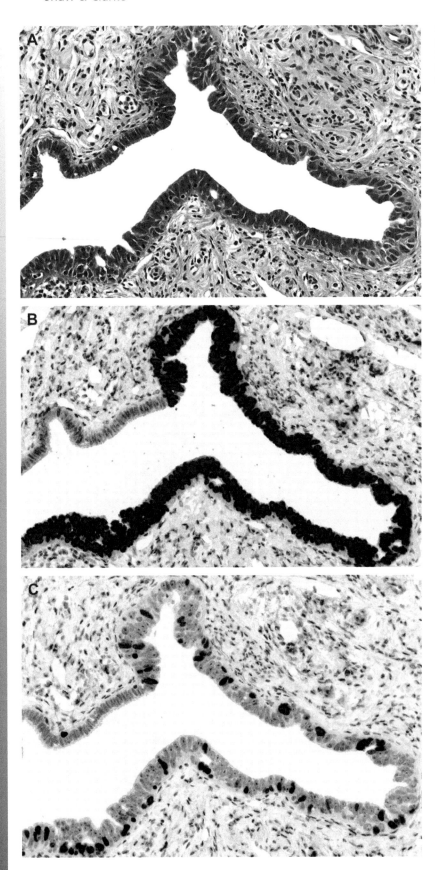

Fig. 5. Serous tubal intraepithelial carcinoma (STIC). (*A*) H&E. (*B*) p53 (diffuse nuclear overexpression). (*C*) Ki67.

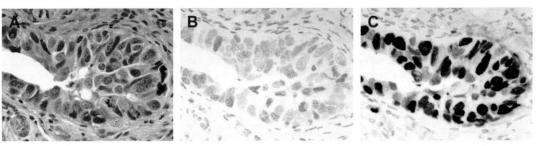

Fig. 6. Serous tubal intraepithelial carcinoma (STIC). (A) H&E. (B) p53 (null pattern of expression). (C) Ki67. (Reprinted from Shaw PA, Rouzbahman M, Pizer ES, et al. Candidate serous cancer precursors in fallopian tube epithelium of BRCA1/2 mutation carriers. Mod Pathol 2009;22(9):1136; with permission.)

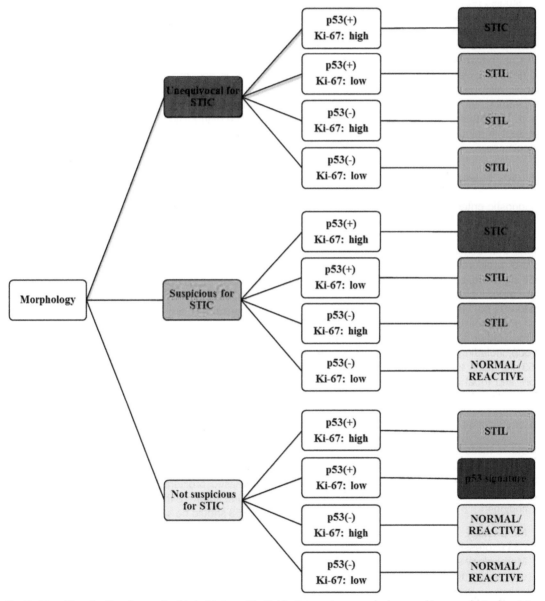

Fig. 7. Algorithm for the diagnosis of tubal intraepithelial lesions, using morphology and immunohistochemistry. Ki67 expression is considered high if positive in at least 10% of lesion cells. p53 is considered positive with either a diffusely positive pattern or a null pattern of expression. Negative p53 in this chart reflects normal, wild-type expression. (Reprinted from Vang R, Visvanathan K, Gross A, et al. Validation of an algorithm for the diagnosis of serous tubal intraepithelial carcinoma. Int J Gynecol Pathol 2012;31(3):243–53; with permission.)

observational, resulting in an overestimate of STIC frequency. The frequency of STIC lesions increases with age and is lower with oral contraceptive use,[49] and this is not controlled for in most publications. STIC is also seen with a lower frequency in women with a strong family history but with negative germline testing. Finally, and importantly, the histologic criteria used to detect the precursor lesions vary from study to study. The inclusion of immunohistochemistry for p53 and Ki67 in the diagnostic algorithm significantly improves the reproducibility of the diagnosis, and the studies reporting a lower frequency have not necessarily followed this approach.[22,32,38,46,50–52] Taking these factors into consideration, the estimate for STIC frequency in BRCA1 mutation carriers is between 5% and 10% and is likely somewhat lower in BRCA2 mutation carriers. It should also be noted that the incidence of STIC in women at no known genetic risk is not zero[22,26,32]; this is an important factor and should be kept in mind when processing salpingectomy specimens.

SEROUS TUBAL INTRAEPITHELIAL LESION

Diagnostic criteria for STIC and for p53 signature incorporate morphology and biomarker interpretation. When using these criteria, there are tubal lesions that demonstrate more features of atypia and/or proliferation than would be expected in a p53 signature, but do not fulfill the criteria required for a reproducible diagnosis of STIC. This group of lesions is not yet well characterized, and the clinical relevance of these lesions is poorly understood. Other terms have been applied to this group, including atypical hyperplasia, proliferative p53 signature, tubal intraepithelial lesion in transition, and tubal atypia, but the authors prefer the designation STIL.

MICROSCOPIC

Because these lesions are not well understood, it is recommended that the STIC diagnostic algorithm be followed. An STIL diagnosis is most commonly made with the following combination of findings:

i. Morphology unequivocal for STIC, abnormal p53 expression, Ki67 less than 10%
ii. Morphology suspicious for STIC, abnormal p53 expression, Ki67 less than 10%

These features indicate that significant alterations have occurred, but that the criteria for a diagnosis of intraepithelial carcinoma are not fulfilled (**Figs. 8** and **9**).

It seems likely, because of the widespread variation of morphologic features and biomarker expression in this group; some of these lesions in fact are benign or reactive changes, not cancer precursors, and others, particularly those STILs with abnormal p53 expression, are cancer precursors with variable transcriptomic/genomic alterations resulting in variable histologic phenotypes. Because of the uncertainty of both diagnostic reproducibility and clinical relevance, some investigators have recommended that a diagnosis of STIL (or proliferative p53 signature) not be used in clinical practice. An alternative to this, which the authors currently practice, is that a lesion with significant atypia and abnormal p53 expression and increased proliferation, but less than the 10% Ki67 index, is diagnosed as STIL. The diagnosis is accompanied by a comment indicating that an atypical lesion of uncertain clinical relevance is present, and that there is no histologic evidence diagnostic of intraepithelial carcinoma.

p53 SIGNATURE

The p53 signature is recognized and diagnosed only after immunohistochemistry for p53 and Ki67 has been performed. There is typically no discernible morphologic lesion on routine examination. p53 signatures are frequent in the fallopian tubes of women at both low and high genetic risk of HGSC, with an incidence of 11% to 46% of resected tubes from women with or without germline mutations, and with and without HGSC.[22,53,54] Because they are seen with a relatively high frequency in premenopausal women with no known genetic predisposition to HGSC, and because, in at least one study, p53 signature is not associated with ovarian cancer risk factors, this lesion may be considered to be a latent cancer precursor.[49,55]

MICROSCOPIC

The p53 signature has been defined as a focus of benign-appearing nonciliated tubal epithelium with nuclear overexpression of p53 but no increased proliferation compared with the background tubal epithelium. Nuclear overexpression of p53 should be seen in a minimum of 12 consecutive cells.[53,56] Although p53 signatures cannot be detected by routine H&E examination alone, once they are detected by immunohistochemistry, the cells of the p53 signature may appear to be distinct from the background tubal epithelium. The cells are nonciliated, with a secretory cell phenotype. Some lesions may have occasional residual ciliated cells. The cells may have minimal atypia compared with background epithelium,

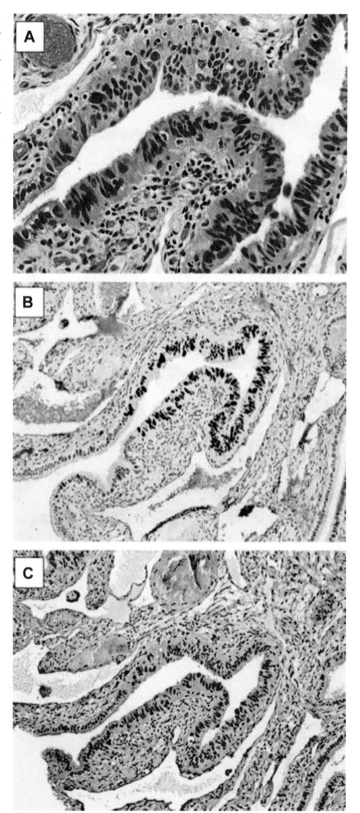

Fig. 8. STIL. (*A*) H&E. (*B*) p53. (*C*) Ki67. Abnormal morphology at least suspicious for STIC, diffuse p53 expression, but no increased Ki67 expression. (*Reprinted from* Visvanathan K, Vang R, Shaw P, et al. Diagnosis of serous tubal intraepithelial carcinoma based on morphologic and immunohistochemical features: a reproducibility study. Am J Surg Pathol 2011;35(12):1772; with permission.)

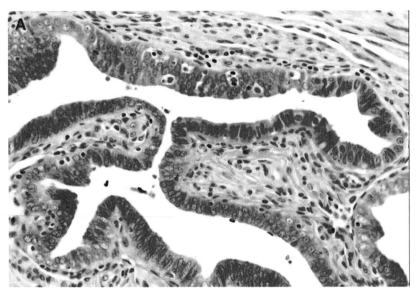

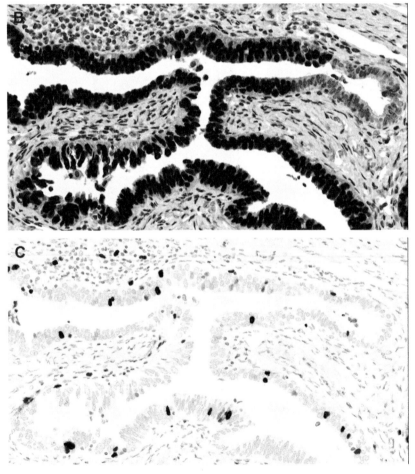

Fig. 9. STIL. (*A*) H&E. (*B*) p53. (*C*) Ki67. Abnormal morphology at least suspicious for STIC, diffuse p53 expression, with increased Ki67 expression that is less than 10% of the lesion cells. (*From* Shaw PA, Clarke B, George S. Precursor lesions of high grade serous carcinoma. In: Fadare O, editor. Precancerous lesions of the gynecologic tract: diagnostic and molecular genetic pathology. Switzerland: Springer International Publishing, 2016; with permission.)

but by definition there are no diagnostic features of malignancy (Fig. 10).

p53 signatures typically involve the tubal fimbria and distal end of the tube. They may be multifocal and bilateral and are seen more frequently in tubes with malignant changes (STIC).[22,53] Other immunohistochemistry stains positive for secretory tubal cells are also expressed in the p53 signature, including PAX8, HMFG2, and CK7.

As might be expected with the intense positive nuclear staining seen in p53 signatures, at least some of these lesions are associated with mutations of the p53 gene.[53] p53 signatures also upregulate phosphorylated γH2AX, a biomarker reflective of concomitant DNA damage (double-strand breaks).[53] The colocalization of p53 signatures with γH2AX suggests that the p53 signature is caused by DNA damage, and that the coexistence of p53 mutations (present in at least some p53 signatures) and unrepaired double-stranded DNA breaks may coexist before malignant transformation.

Currently, p53 signatures are usually not reported clinically.

DIFFERENTIAL DIAGNOSIS

The differential diagnosis includes metastatic spread of HGSC, metastases from non-tubo-ovarian sites, metaplastic changes, hyperplasias, and benign tumorlike lesions.

The recognition, description, and molecular/genetic analyses of STICs are extremely important in furthering the understanding of how HGSC begins and will influence future preventative and early detection strategies. Care must be taken however in the interpretation of tubal lesions in the setting of HGSC resection specimens. It is possible that lesions that are consistent with STIC may in fact be peritoneal/mucosal spread from HGSC tumor. Although considered to be rare, mucosal implants on the tubal fimbria from nongynecologic cancers do occur, and it is possible that some cases of apparent STIC may represent spread, not origin, from an ovarian tumor.[57] It is currently not possible using standard technologies to differentiated STIC from intramucosal spread from HGSC.

Metastases have been reported from various sites, with most being adenocarcinomas from colon, breast, or endocervix (Fig. 11). Lymphoma, neuroendocrine tumors, and mesotheliomas may also involve the fallopian tube. Most of the metastatic tumors will be readily identified by the presence of tumor elsewhere in the tube, gynecologic tract, and/or peritoneum. The tubal involvement includes submucosa, muscularis, serosa, lumen, lymphovascular spaces, with only a few being restricted to fimbrial mucosa. The histomorphology is usually readily distinguishable, but immunohistochemistry may be required to distinguish a metastasis from a de novo tubal intraepithelial carcinoma, which involves only the tubal epithelium.

Transitional cell metaplasia of tubal epithelium is commonly seen and is readily distinguished from STIC with a flat architecture and low-grade nuclei. Walthard nests have longitudinally grooved bland nuclei. Mucinous metaplasia (Fig. 12) is occasionally seen and may be associated with Peutz-Jeghers syndrome.

Epithelial hyperplasia is not usually associated with cytologic atypia, but reactive epithelial changes may be present when associated with marked chronic inflammation, and this may result in confusion with a malignant process, especially in the presence of florid salpingitis. Papillary tubal hyperplasia has been described recently and may be a precursor of serous borderline tumors of the ovary (Fig. 13).[58] Reactive changes associated with inflammation and hyperplasia will have a mix of secretory and ciliated cells. Immunohistochemistry for p53 will be within normal limits (wild-type pattern) in hyperplasia.

Secretory cell outgrowths (SCOUT), considered by some to be a benign latent cancer precursor, is

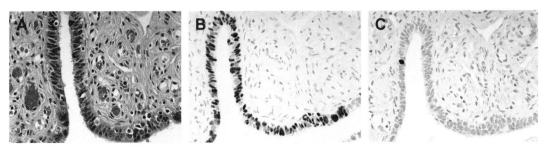

Fig. 10. p53 signature. (*A*) H&E. (*B*) p53. (*C*) Ki67. (*Reprinted from* Shaw PA, Rouzbahman M, Pizer ES, et al. Candidate serous cancer precursors in fallopian tube epithelium of BRCA1/2 mutation carriers. Mod Pathol 2009;22(9):1135; with permission.)

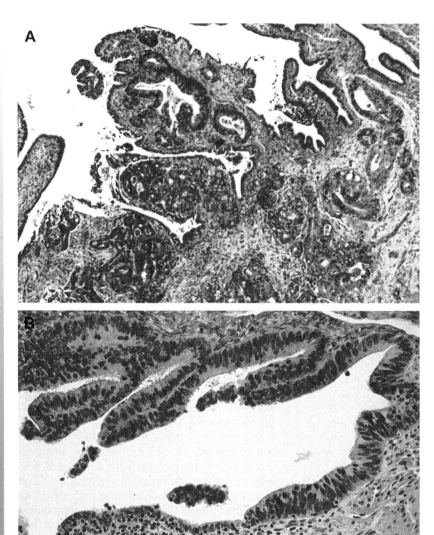

Fig. 11. Metastatic carcinoma to the tubal mucosa. (*A*) Colorectal carcinoma, (*B*) Endocervical carcinoma.

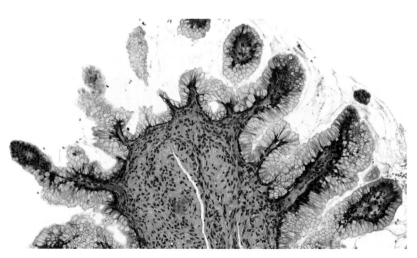

Fig. 12. Mucinous metaplasia of tubal epithelium.

Fig. 13. Papillary tubal metaplasia.

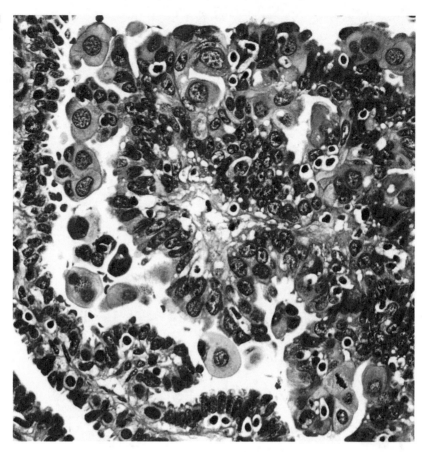

a focus of secretory cells without, or with very few, intervening ciliated cells (**Fig. 14**).[56,59] SCOUTs are present throughout the length of the fallopian tube and often stand out from the normal adjacent epithelium with greater pseudostratification and columnar alignment of cells. They are seen more commonly in association with HGSC, but when present alone, have little diagnostic significance. SCOUTs do not have cytologic atypia, do not have increased proliferation compared with background tubal epithelium, and do not overexpress p53.

Extraovarian sex-cord proliferations of the tube have a characteristic histomorphology, have minimal atypia, and express inhibin (**Fig. 15**).[60]

LYNCH SYNDROME

The authors recently reviewed their experience with prophylactic samples from 25 LS patients.[61] They found an 8% (2/25) incidence of carcinoma: both cases were of endometrioid histology and early stage (1A). Six cases (24%) showed atypical hyperplasia/endometrial intraepithelial neoplasia without associated carcinoma. The authors' data are similar to the Memorial Sloan Kettering review

of prophylactic specimens in LS patients.[62] They similarly showed a 24% incidence of endometrial endometrioid carcinoma or its precursor lesions (2 patients with early-stage FIGO [International Federation of Gynecology and Obstetrics] grade 1 endometrioid endometrial carcinomas and 3 patients with atypical hyperplasia, unassociated with carcinoma). One patient was found to have a mixed endometrioid/clear cell OC.

All cell types of endometrial cancer have been implicated in LS but with endometrioid subtype being the most common. Similarly, in review of findings of prophylactic hysterectomy specimens in LS patients, most cases of incidental carcinoma are of endometrioid histology, but there have been single case reports of type 2 endometrial cancers identified in prophylactic specimens from LS patients. Palma and colleagues[63] identified a high-grade endometrial cancer and a synchronous mixed clear cell and endometrioid primary fallopian tube carcinoma in an MSH2 patient at 51 years of age. Chung and colleagues[64] identified a mixed clear cell and endometrioid carcinoma of endometrium in a 48-year-old MSH2 carrier.

Table 1 summarizes the cancer findings in prophylactic gynecologic specimens from LS

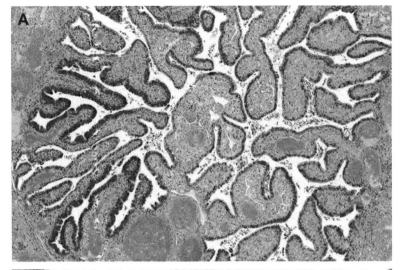

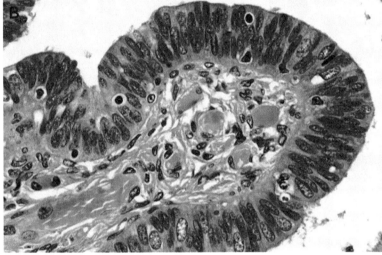

Fig. 14. SCOUT. (*A*) Cross-section of midportion of fallopian tube. SCOUTs stand out as darker ribbons of epithelium (*left side* of photograph). (*B*) SCOUT epithelium appears stratified, with columnar cells and elongated columnar nuclei. Rare residual ciliated cells may be present.

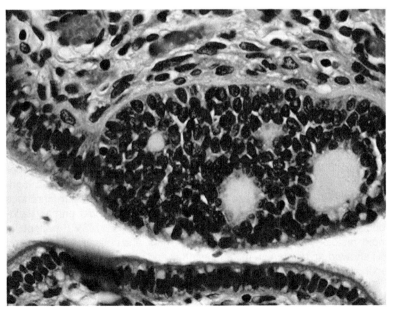

Fig. 15. Extraovarian sex-cord proliferation at distal end of fallopian tube.

Table 1
Malignant and premalignant findings in prophylactic gynecologic specimens from Lynch syndrome carriers

Study	Age	Gene	Stage	Tumor 1	Tumor 2	Tumor Seen at Time of Grossing
Palma et al,[63] 2008	51	MSH2	—	Mixed clear cell endometrioid PFTC	High-grade endometrial cancer, NOS	No
Mills et al,[65] 2012	NA	Known LS	NA	EC-LUS	—	NA
Mills et al,[65] 2012	NA	Known LS	NA	Endocervical carcinoma, but MMR-IHC intact	—	NA
Downes et al,[61] 2014 (case 1)	47	MLH1	NA	CAH	—	No
Downes et al,[61] 2014 (case 4)	43	MSH2	NA	CAH	—	No
Downes et al,[61] 2014 (case 8)	42	MSH2	pT1a	EC grade 1	—	Yes
Downes et al,[61] 2014 (case 15)	44	MLH1	NA	CAH	—	No
Downes et al,[61] 2014 (case 16)	50	MSH2	NA	CAH	—	Yes
Downes et al,[61] 2014 (case 18)	50	MSH6	NA	CAH	—	No
Downes et al,[61] 2014 (case 22)	59	MSH6	pT1a	EC grade 2	—	Yes
Downes et al,[61] 2014 (case 23)	48	MSH2	NA	CAH	—	No
Chung et al,[64] 2003	48	MSH2	pT1b	Mixed clear and endometrioid-LUS	—	—
Schmeler et al,[66] 2006	38, 58, 48	NA	2 stage 1 and one stage 2	EC-NOS	—	NA
Pistorius et al,[67] 2006	49	Unknown	pT1b	EC-NOS	—	NA
Pistorius et al,[67] 2006	47	MSH2	pT1b	EC-NOS	—	NA
Karamurzin et al,[62] 2013	54	MSH2	pT1a	EC grade 1	—	NA
Karamurzin et al,[62] 2013	56	MLH1	pT1a	EC grade 1	—	NA
Karamurzin et al,[62] 2013	35	MLH1	NA	CAH	—	NA
Karamurzin et al,[62] 2013	45	MLH1	NA	CAH	—	NA
Karamurzin et al,[62] 2013	53	MSH2	NA	CAH	—	NA
Karamurzin et al,[62] 2013	44	MSH2	—	Ovary-clear/ endometrioid	—	NA

Abbreviations: CAH, complex atypical hyperplasia; EC, endometrial carcinoma; IHC, immunohistochemistry; LUS, lower uterine segment; NA, not available; NOS, not otherwise specified; PFTC, primary fallopian tube carcinoma.

patients, including histologic subtypes, gene affected, and patient age.[61–67]

Currently, it is recommended that women identified as being at genetic risk for LS-associated endometrial and ovarian cancer undergo annual gynecologic examination, pelvic ultrasound, and endometrial biopsy beginning between ages 30 and 35 years. Prophylactic hysterectomy and bilateral salpingo-oophorectomy should be considered when child-bearing is completed.[68]

For LS patients undergoing prophylactic gynecologic surgery, the authors recommend performing an endometrial biopsy before surgery, to rule out an unexpected cancer to ensure patients undergo preoperative workup and, if necessary, full staging.

In the authors' audit of 25 cases of prophylactic hysterectomy specimens from LS patients, they noted a lack of consistency in grossing of such specimens. They attempted to derive recommendations but acknowledge that the data are limited. In their center, for such cases they submit endometrium and lower uterine segment in toto. The latter is predicated on the work of Westin and colleagues, who showed a strong association between location of EC in LUS and LS.[69] Furthermore, they apply the SEE-FIM protocol for processing tubes and ovaries in such cases, although HGSC is not part of the syndrome. Processing of the nonfimbrial end of the tube in toto is important because an incidental primary tubal carcinoma has been described. Should a patient undergoing such surgery have an ovarian mass, representative sections are suggested based on the gross assessment of the lesion.

REFERENCES

1. Walsh T, Casadei S, Lee MK, et al. Mutations in 12 genes for inherited ovarian, fallopian tube, and peritoneal carcinoma identified by massively parallel sequencing. Proc Natl Acad Sci U S A 2011; 108(44):18032–7.

2. Shaw PA, McLaughlin JR, Zweemer RP, et al. Histopathologic features of genetically determined ovarian cancer. Int J Gynecol Pathol 2002;21(4):407–11.

3. Cancer Genome Atlas Research Network. Integrated genomic analyses of ovarian carcinoma. Nature 2011;474(7353):609–15.

4. Ramus SJ, Song H, Dicks E, et al. Germline mutations in the BRIP1, BARD1, PALB2, and NBN genes in women with ovarian cancer. J Natl Cancer Inst 2015;107(11).

5. Domchek SM, Friebel TM, Singer CF, et al. Association of risk-reducing surgery in BRCA1 or BRCA2 mutation carriers with cancer risk and mortality. JAMA 2010;304(9):967–75.

6. Greene MH, Piedmonte M, Alberts D, et al. A prospective study of risk-reducing salpingo-oophorectomy and longitudinal CA-125 screening among women at increased genetic risk of ovarian cancer: design and baseline characteristics: a Gynecologic Oncology Group study. Cancer Epidemiol Biomarkers Prev 2008;17(3):594–604.

7. Walker JL, Powell CB, Chen LM, et al. Society of Gynecologic Oncology recommendations for the prevention of ovarian cancer. Cancer 2015;121(13): 2108–20.

8. Lu KH, Dinh M, Kohlmann W, et al. Gynecologic cancer as a "sentinel cancer" for women with hereditary nonpolyposis colorectal cancer syndrome. Obstet Gynecol 2005;105(3):569–74.

9. Boland CR, Shike M. Report from the Jerusalem workshop on Lynch syndrome—hereditary nonpolyposis colorectal cancer. Gastroenterology 2010; 138(7):2197.e1–7.

10. Ferguson SE, Aronson M, Pollett A, et al. Performance characteristics of screening strategies for Lynch syndrome in unselected women with newly diagnosed endometrial cancer who have undergone universal germline mutation testing. Cancer 2014; 120(24):3932–9.

11. Beamer LC, Grant ML, Espenschied CR, et al. Reflex immunohistochemistry and microsatellite instability testing of colorectal tumors for Lynch syndrome among US cancer programs and follow-up of abnormal results. J Clin Oncol 2012; 30(10):1058–63.

12. Chui MH, Ryan P, Radigan J, et al. The histomorphology of Lynch syndrome-associated ovarian carcinomas: toward a subtype-specific screening strategy. Am J Surg Pathol 2014;38(9):1173–81.

13. Le DT, Uram JN, Wang H, et al. PD-1 blockade in tumors with mismatch-repair deficiency. N Engl J Med 2015;372(26):2509–20.

14. Ladabaum U, Wang G, Terdiman J, et al. Strategies to identify the Lynch syndrome among patients with colorectal cancer: a cost-effectiveness analysis. Ann Intern Med 2011;155(2):69–79.

15. Tan MH, Mester JL, Ngeow J, et al. Lifetime cancer risks in individuals with germline PTEN mutations. Clin Cancer Res 2012;18(2):400–7.

16. Piek JM, van Diest PJ, Zweemer RP, et al. Dysplastic changes in prophylactically removed Fallopian tubes of women predisposed to developing ovarian cancer. J Pathol 2001;195(4):451–6.

17. Shaw P, Rouzbahman M, Murphy J, et al. Mucosal epithelial proliferation and p53 overexpression are frequent in women with BRCA mutations. Mod Pathol 2004;17(Supp 1):214A.

18. Finch A, Shaw P, Rosen B, et al. Clinical and pathologic findings of prophylactic salpingo-oophorectomies in 159 BRCA1 and BRCA2 carriers. Gynecol Oncol 2006;100(1):58–64.

19. Medeiros F, Muto MG, Lee Y, et al. The tubal fimbria is a preferred site for early adenocarcinoma in women with familial ovarian cancer syndrome. Am J Surg Pathol 2006;30(2):230–6.

20. Crum CP, Drapkin R, Miron A, et al. The distal fallopian tube: a new model for pelvic serous carcinogenesis. Curr Opin Obstet Gynecol 2007;19(1):3–9.

21. Jarboe E, Folkins A, Nucci MR, et al. Serous carcinogenesis in the fallopian tube: a descriptive classification. Int J Gynecol Pathol 2008;27(1):1–9.

22. Shaw PA, Rouzbahman M, Pizer ES, et al. Candidate serous cancer precursors in fallopian tube epithelium of BRCA1/2 mutation carriers. Mod Pathol 2009;22(9):1133–8.

23. McAlpine JN, Hanley GE, Woo MM, et al. Opportunistic salpingectomy: uptake, risks, and complications of a regional initiative for ovarian cancer prevention. Am J Obstet Gynecol 2014;210(5): 471.e1–11.

24. Greene MH, Mai PL. The fallopian tube: from back stage to center stage. Cancer Prev Res (Phila) 2015;8(5):339–41.

25. Longacre TA, Oliva E, Soslow RA, Association of Directors of Anatomic and Surgical Pathology. Recommendations for the reporting of fallopian tube neoplasms. Hum Pathol 2007;38(8):1160–3.

26. Rabban JT, Garg K, Crawford B, et al. Early detection of high-grade tubal serous carcinoma in women at low risk for hereditary breast and ovarian cancer syndrome by systematic examination of fallopian tubes incidentally removed during benign surgery. Am J Surg Pathol 2014;38(6):729–42.

27. Rabban JT, Krasik E, Chen LM, et al. Multistep level sections to detect occult fallopian tube carcinoma in risk-reducing salpingo-oophorectomies from women with BRCA mutations: implications for defining an optimal specimen dissection protocol. Am J Surg Pathol 2009;33(12):1878–85.

28. Colgan TJ, Murphy J, Cole DE, et al. Occult carcinoma in prophylactic oophorectomy specimens: prevalence and association with BRCA germline mutation status. Am J Surg Pathol 2001;25(10): 1283–9.

29. Powell CB, Kenley E, Chen LM, et al. Risk-reducing salpingo-oophorectomy in BRCA mutation carriers: role of serial sectioning in the detection of occult malignancy. J Clin Oncol 2005;23(1):127–32.

30. Rebbeck TR, Lynch HT, Neuhausen SL, et al. Prophylactic oophorectomy in carriers of BRCA1 or BRCA2 mutations. N Engl J Med 2002;346(21): 1616–22.

31. Finch A, Beiner M, Lubinski J, et al. Salpingo-oophorectomy and the risk of ovarian, fallopian tube, and peritoneal cancers in women with a BRCA1 or BRCA2 mutation. JAMA 2006;296(2):185–92.

32. Sherman ME, Piedmonte M, Mai PL, et al. Pathologic findings at risk-reducing salpingo-oophorectomy: primary results from Gynecologic Oncology Group Trial GOG-0199. J Clin Oncol 2014;32(29):3275–83.

33. Powell CB, Chen LM, McLennan J, et al. Risk-reducing salpingo-oophorectomy (RRSO) in BRCA mutation carriers: experience with a consecutive series of 111 patients using a standardized surgical-pathological protocol. Int J Gynecol Cancer 2011; 21(5):846–51.

34. Finch AP, Lubinski J, Moller P, et al. Impact of oophorectomy on cancer incidence and mortality in women with a BRCA1 or BRCA2 mutation. J Clin Oncol 2014;32(15):1547–53.

35. Manchanda R, Abdelraheim A, Johnson M, et al. Outcome of risk-reducing salpingo-oophorectomy in BRCA carriers and women of unknown mutation status. BJOG 2011;118(7):814–24.

36. Powell CB, Swisher EM, Cass I, et al. Long term follow up of BRCA1 and BRCA2 mutation carriers with unsuspected neoplasia identified at risk reducing salpingo-oophorectomy. Gynecol Oncol 2013;129(2):364–71.

37. Nik NN, Vang R, Shih Ie M, et al. Origin and pathogenesis of pelvic (ovarian, tubal, and primary peritoneal) serous carcinoma. Annu Rev Pathol 2014;9: 27–45.

38. Vang R, Visvanathan K, Gross A, et al. Validation of an algorithm for the diagnosis of serous tubal intraepithelial carcinoma. Int J Gynecol Pathol 2012; 31(3):243–53.

39. Bannatyne P, Russell P. Early adenocarcinoma of the fallopian tubes. A case for multifocal tumorigenesis. Diagn Gynecol Obstet 1981;3(1):49–60.

40. Yanai-Inbar I, Silverberg SG. Mucosal epithelial proliferation of the fallopian tube: prevalence, clinical associations, and optimal strategy for histopathologic assessment. Int J Gynecol Pathol 2000;19(2): 139–44.

41. Kuhn E, Kurman RJ, Vang R, et al. TP53 mutations in serous tubal intraepithelial carcinoma and concurrent pelvic high-grade serous carcinoma–evidence supporting the clonal relationship of the two lesions. J Pathol 2012;226(3):421–6.

42. Kindelberger DW, Lee Y, Miron A, et al. Intraepithelial carcinoma of the fimbria and pelvic serous carcinoma: evidence for a causal relationship. Am J Surg Pathol 2007;31(2):161–9.

43. Przybycin CG, Kurman RJ, Ronnett BM, et al. Are all pelvic (nonuterine) serous carcinomas of tubal origin? Am J Surg Pathol 2010;34(10):1407–16.

44. Tang S, Onuma K, Deb P, et al. Frequency of serous tubal intraepithelial carcinoma in various gynecologic malignancies: a study of 300 consecutive cases. Int J Gynecol Pathol 2012;31(2):103–10.

45. Carlson JW, Jarboe EA, Kindelberger D, et al. Serous tubal intraepithelial carcinoma: diagnostic reproducibility and its implications. Int J Gynecol Pathol 2010;29(4):310–4.

46. Visvanathan K, Vang R, Shaw P, et al. Diagnosis of serous tubal intraepithelial carcinoma based on morphologic and immunohistochemical features: a reproducibility study. Am J Surg Pathol 2011; 35(12):1766–75.

47. Singh N, Gilks CB, Wilkinson N, et al. Assignment of primary site in high-grade serous tubal, ovarian and peritoneal carcinoma: a proposal. Histopathology 2014;65(2):149–54.

48. Wethington SL, Park KJ, Soslow RA, et al. Clinical outcome of isolated serous tubal intraepithelial carcinomas (STIC). Int J Gynecol Cancer 2013;23(9): 1603–11.

49. Vicus D, Shaw PA, Finch A, et al. Risk factors for non-invasive lesions of the fallopian tube in BRCA mutation carriers. Gynecol Oncol 2010;118(3):295–8.

50. Powell CB. Risk reducing salpingo-oophorectomy for BRCA mutation carriers: twenty years later. Gynecol Oncol 2014;132(2):261–3.

51. Mingels MJ, Roelofsen T, van der Laak JA, et al. Tubal epithelial lesions in salpingo-oophorectomy specimens of BRCA-mutation carriers and controls. Gynecol Oncol 2012;127(1):88–93.

52. Reitsma W, de Bock GH, Oosterwijk JC, et al. Clinicopathologic characteristics and survival in BRCA1- and BRCA2-related adnexal cancer: are they different? Int J Gynecol Cancer 2012;22(4):579–85.

53. Lee Y, Miron A, Drapkin R, et al. A candidate precursor to serous carcinoma that originates in the distal fallopian tube. J Pathol 2007;211(1):26–35.

54. Norquist BM, Garcia RL, Allison KH, et al. The molecular pathogenesis of hereditary ovarian carcinoma: alterations in the tubal epithelium of women with BRCA1 and BRCA2 mutations. Cancer 2010; 116(22):5261–71.

55. Crum CP, Herfs M, Ning G, et al. Through the glass darkly: intraepithelial neoplasia, top-down differentiation, and the road to ovarian cancer. J Pathol 2013; 231(4):402–12.

56. Mehrad M, Ning G, Chen EY, et al. A pathologist's road map to benign, precancerous, and malignant intraepithelial proliferations in the fallopian tube. Adv Anat Pathol 2010;17(5):293–302.

57. Rabban JT, Vohra P, Zaloudek CJ. Nongynecologic metastases to fallopian tube mucosa: a potential mimic of tubal high-grade serous carcinoma and benign tubal mucinous metaplasia or nonmucinous hyperplasia. Am J Surg Pathol 2015;39(1):35–51.

58. Kurman RJ, Vang R, Junge J, et al. Papillary tubal hyperplasia: the putative precursor of ovarian atypical proliferative (borderline) serous tumors, noninvasive implants, and endosalpingiosis. Am J Surg Pathol 2011;35(11):1605–14.

59. Chen EY, Mehra K, Mehrad M, et al. Secretory cell outgrowth, PAX2 and serous carcinogenesis in the Fallopian tube. J Pathol 2010;222(1):110–6.

60. McCluggage WG, Stewart CJ, Iacobelli J, et al. Microscopic extraovarian sex cord proliferations: an undescribed phenomenon. Histopathology 2015;66(4):555–64.

61. Downes MR, Allo G, McCluggage WG, et al. Review of findings in prophylactic gynaecological specimens in Lynch syndrome with literature review and recommendations for grossing. Histopathology 2014;65(2):228–39.

62. Karamurzin Y, Soslow RA, Garg K. Histologic evaluation of prophylactic hysterectomy and oophorectomy in Lynch syndrome. Am J Surg Pathol 2013; 37(4):579–85.

63. Palma L, Marcus V, Gilbert L, et al. Synchronous occult cancers of the endometrium and fallopian tube in an MSH2 mutation carrier at time of prophylactic surgery. Gynecol Oncol 2008;111(3):575–8.

64. Chung L, Broaddus R, Crozier M, et al. Unexpected endometrial cancer at prophylactic hysterectomy in a woman with hereditary nonpolyposis colon cancer. Obstet Gynecol 2003;102(5 Pt 2):1152–5.

65. Mills AM, Liou S, Kong CS, et al. Are women with endocervical adenocarcinoma at risk for Lynch syndrome? Evaluation of 101 cases including unusual subtypes and lower uterine segment tumors. Int J Gynecol Pathol 2012;31(5):463–9.

66. Schmeler KM, Lynch HT, Chen LM, et al. Prophylactic surgery to reduce the risk of gynecologic cancers in the Lynch syndrome. N Engl J Med 2006;354(3): 261–9.

67. Pistorius S, Kruger S, Hohl R, et al. Occult endometrial cancer and decision making for prophylactic hysterectomy in hereditary nonpolyposis colorectal cancer patients. Gynecol Oncol 2006;102(2): 189–94.

68. Stoffel EM, Mangu PB, Gruber SB, et al. Hereditary colorectal cancer syndromes: American Society of Clinical Oncology Clinical Practice Guideline endorsement of the familial risk-colorectal cancer: European Society for Medical Oncology Clinical Practice Guidelines. J Clin Oncol 2015;33(2): 209–17.

69. Westin SN, Lacour RA, Urbauer DL, et al. Carcinoma of the lower uterine segment: a newly described association with Lynch syndrome. J Clin Oncol 2008; 26(36):5965–71.

Image Analysis in Surgical Pathology

Mark C. Lloyd, PhD[a,b,*], James P. Monaco, PhD[c], Marilyn M. Bui, MD, PhD[d,*]

KEYWORDS

- Image analysis • Surgical pathology • Digital pathology

ABSTRACT

Digitization of glass slides of surgical pathology samples facilitates a number of value-added capabilities beyond what a pathologist could previously do with a microscope. Image analysis is one of the most fundamental opportunities to leverage the advantages that digital pathology provides. The ability to quantify aspects of a digital image is an extraordinary opportunity to collect data with exquisite accuracy and reliability. In this review, we describe the history of image analysis in pathology and the present state of technology processes as well as examples of research and clinical use.

OVERVIEW

Image analysis is a method by which meaningful information is extracted from a digital image.[1] By its very nature, image analysis is a reproducible and objective way to quantify a specific aspect of some feature that exists in a sample. This could be the intensity of a staining pattern or the size of a nucleus. In fact, it can be far more complex.

Image analysis is a general term that is not specific to digital pathology. In fact, digital pathology is one of the most recent major medical applications for a concept incepted since the 1940s and 1950s when computer usages in medicine first began to emerge. The growth of image analysis has been considerable in the past 3 to 4 decades as computers have become far more accessible and file storage continues to get less expensive.[2] Well over 100,000 published peer-reviewed articles address medical image analysis (**Fig. 1**). It is clear that in the 1980s image analysis was becoming more accessible. This was due in large part to the expansion of image analysis into radiology. Over the course of the past 2 decades, a new family of image analysis tools has clearly emerged for pathology.[3] In this review, we focus on the emergence of image analysis for surgical or anatomic pathology.

In 1997, a comprehensive review was published by Meijer and colleagues[4] that describes the 3 most general and inclusive areas of image analysis, including (1) morphometry, the measure of geometric features; (2) quantification/counting, the measure of the number of objects; and (3) cytometry/pattern recognition, the measure of cellular features (ie, chromatin). Since the late 1990s, a considerable amount of literature has focused on digital pathology image analysis, and a number of commercial products have become available.

Image analysis was first performed in pathology using cameras mounted in the light path of a standard clinical or research-grade microscope. However, today, high-throughput slide scanning instruments are available. Slide scanners made a considerable mark on the history of image analysis of histologic samples. Slide scanning brought technical and accessibility advantages to the field. By controlling and calibrating the light sources and flattening the background, these instruments produce relatively homogeneous images. Furthermore, by producing whole slide images (WSIs), the pathologist is no longer limited to specific fields of view. Finally, the increasing speed of acquisition of these instruments is bringing a digital pathology workflow to those institutions that are the earliest adopters. In summary, slide scanning technology has facilitated the enhanced the utility of image analysis for pathology considerably. Although some technical, regulatory, societal, and other

[a] Analytic Microscopy Core, H. Lee Moffitt Cancer Center and Research Institute, Tampa, FL, USA; [b] Department of Biological Sciences, University of Chicago Illinois, 845 West Taylor Street, Chicago, IL 60607, USA; [c] Inspirata, Inc. Tampa, FL, USA; [d] Analytic Microscopy Core, Department of Anatomic Pathology, H. Lee Moffitt Cancer Center and Research Institute, 12902 Magnolia Drive, Tampa, FL 33612, USA
* Corresponding author. H. Lee Moffitt Cancer Center and Research Institute, 12902 Magnolia Drive, SRB-4, Tampa, FL 33612.
E-mail addresses: mlloyd8@uic.edu; marilyn.bui@moffitt.org

Surgical Pathology 9 (2016) 329–337
http://dx.doi.org/10.1016/j.path.2016.02.001

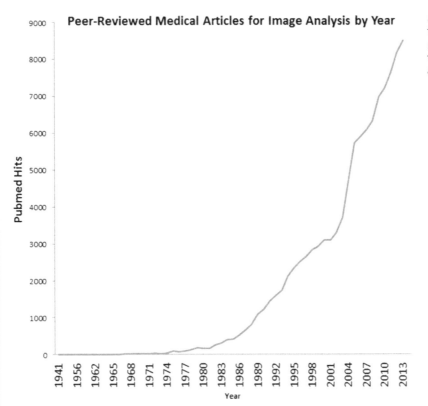

Peer-Reviewed Medical Articles for Image Analysis by Year

Fig. 1. Peer-reviewed articles available on www.pubmed.gov by year for the search term "image analysis."

challenges remain, the future is bright for image analysis of surgical pathology specimens.

PROCESSES

The routine surgical pathology specimens that are subject to microscopic examination are glass slides with a surface 3 to 4 micro-slices of formalin-fixed and paraffin-embedded tissue sections with various stains including hematoxylin-eosin stain (H&E), immunohistochemical-based stain (IHC), and special chemical stains. Fluorescence-based stain is less frequently used for clinical specimens but common for research specimens. The process of analyzing an image for surgical pathology specimens begins after the image is acquired. The images include the whole slide, portion of the slide, or static images of specific areas of interest. Image acquisition alone does not include image management, image query, or image sharing or related digital pathology subjects. This can, at times, be confusing because commercially available tools often provide a complete digital pathology workflow solution. Image acquisition to archive quality images is the single most important step toward achieving meaningful image analysis result. Issues related to image acquisition will be discussed elsewhere in this issue. For the purposes of this review, we divided the image analysis section into 3 main categories after image acquisition: (1) segmentation, (2) classification, and (3) results. Within each of these 3 categories we address morphometry, counting, and color/texture. This is a massive oversimplification of the utility of image analysis for pathology; however, the goal is to describe in enough detail, for a broad audience, how image analysis can work using surgical pathology specimens.

IMAGE SEGMENTATION

Segmentation is a method for dividing an image into smaller subsegments. By segmenting an image, one can break the image into similar pieces that can then be evaluated in a more meaningful way (**Fig. 2**). Segmentation can be completed using a number of different methods. It is not our goal to describe the advantages or disadvantages of any particular method, or even to create a comprehensive list of methods. Our goal is to describe, in general terms, the depth and breadth of opportunities to parse an image into smaller pieces using the methodology most likely to yield the desired results. For example, well over a dozen families of image segmentation methodologies exist for pathology images. Given the multitude of different techniques, we have chosen a subset

Fig. 2. Segmentation example across the WSI (scale = 5 mm) and individual nuclei (scale = 250 µm).

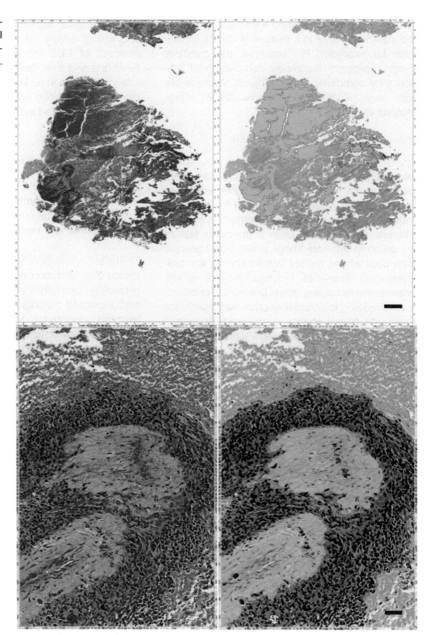

of the 7 most common segmentation schemas for pathology images to date. These methods continue to advance rapidly, and investigators interested in the latest segmentation technologies should consult recent literature.

The methods that are described at a high level include (1) simple splitting geometries or split and merge techniques; (2) thresholding, watershedding, or histogram-based techniques; (3) clustering; (4) edge detection; (5) partial differentiation equation (PDE)-based; (6) graph partitioning; and (7) trainable techniques.

Splitting

At its most basic, splitting divides an image into halves, quadrants, or equal-sized squares (eg, checkerboard).[5] The granularity of the checkerboard determines the fineness of the segmentation. The largest number of objects can be created by using the checkerboard with objects that are the size of 1 pixel (which tends to be unnecessarily computationally expensive). As simplistic as this technique first appears, it can become complex as small objects (single pixel, for example) are recombined if they are neighbors and sufficiently alike in a feature of choice (similar color for example). For example, the quadtree merging process enhances computational efficiency by combining similar objects so fewer objects must be evaluated in downstream image analysis steps.[6]

Thresholding, Watershedding, and/or Histogram-Based Techniques

Here we have combined at least 3 families of segmentation methods into one. Although a gross oversimplification, this allows us to focus on the underlying technique of each method as a single rationale. Thresholding uses a specified feature (eg, color) to separate image pixels into 2 groups: each pixel whose feature value exceeds the predetermined threshold belongs in one group, whereas the remaining pixels belong in the other.[7] Watershedding is a transformation that thresholds pixels into binary groups using gradient magnitudes (ie, the slope of the image surface).[8] Where large gradients exist, threshold lines are defined. Histogram-based techniques use the values of a given feature (eg, color) and histogram shape (eg, peaks and valleys) to determine appropriate thresholds for segmenting the pixels.

Clustering

The most prominently used clustering method, K-means, is an algorithm that first chooses cluster centers and then groups each pixel with the closest cluster center. Note that K-means operates in a specified feature space (eg, RGB color space); thus, 2 points that are close in a spatial sense may not be close in the chosen feature space.[9] Although there are many ways to determine the cluster seed point (center), the concept of grouping pixels into objects by likeness for a given feature is the distinguishing concept.

Edge Detection

This segmentation method identifies boundaries within an image (ie, color changes).[10] The boundaries, or edges, are found at regions of intense or sharp variation. In many ways, edge detection is similar to thresholding and watershedding; however, the most significant difference is that (depending on the detection method) the edges may not form closed boundaries; that is, they can have holes. Thus, region segmentation may require ancillary algorithms capable of filling in the gaps.

Partial-Differential Equations

A number of PDE models exist; for example, active contour models. Although the mathematics of

each individual algorithm can be rather complex and out of scope for this overview, the general concept of PDE models is using multivariable functions and their partial derivatives to establish rates of change in an image. When contours or regions are identified within an image, the image may be segmented into objects.[11]

Graph Partitioning

By considering image pixels as nodes on a graph, the graph-partitioning algorithms may segment the pixels into groups. A number of popular graph-partitioning methods are used in pathology image segmentation today, including the spanning-tree and random walker methods.[12]

Trainable Techniques

Image segmentation may also be completed by providing computer learning algorithms with input and expected outputs.[13] By using the computer learning algorithms to evaluate and process optimal paths for further segmentation, an unsupervised segmentation is possible. Neural networks of many kinds are an ideal example of trainable segmentation methods that take into account far more parameters than the single or small groups of features discussed in any of the prior segmentation methods. Neural networks, for example, may be used to create decision-making mechanisms far more complex than traditional methods.

In summary, many segmentation methods exist. The purpose of each segmentation method is to parse large objects into smaller objects that have similar features. This allows the image analyst to be able to group segments for classification.

STATISTICAL CLASSIFICATION

Classification methods are used to assign meaning to the objects that were previously segmented. The purpose of classification is to use contextual information provided by the segmentation (ie, similar color intensity) to assign segments into groups (**Fig. 3**). Similar to segmentation, several methodologies for classification exist and the field continues to innovate novel classification techniques. It is also worth noting that the difference between segmentation and classification is sometimes unclear. For the purposes of this review, classification is the assignment of objects to categorize the objects.

Rather than go into the details of several mathematically complex classification methods, we simply list and briefly describe the concepts of some of the most prominent classifiers used in pathology image analysis. These classifiers include (1) Markov chains and Markov meshes, (2) Naive Bayes classifiers, (3)

Fig. 3. Classification example for separating groups of objects by specific characteristics.

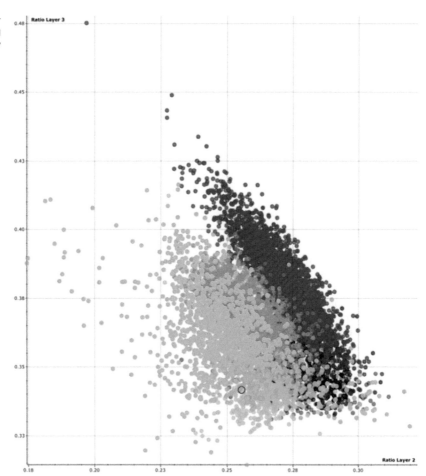

support vector machines (SVMs), (4) logistic regression, and (4) random forest classifiers.

Markov Chains and Markov Meshes

Markov chains, field models, and meshes are mathematical methodologies that may be applied to histologic images for classification.[14] Although entire books have been written on the Markov approaches to image analysis, we simply intend on introducing the idea of using statistical tools to classify large data sets, such as WSIs. Very generally speaking, Markov methods work by sampling the probability distributions in a sequential fashion, a chain for example, transitioning from state to state within a certain probability.

Naive Bayes Classifiers

Another statistical family of classifiers, Naive Bayes classifiers, are probabilistic and assume all features are unrelated; that is, each feature (eg, color, shape) is considered independently.[15]

Support Vector Machines

Supervised (manual interaction) machine learning algorithms, including SVM, are becoming increasingly common in modern image classification of WSIs.[16] Here, pattern recognition is used to classify objects. It is considered supervised when a user trains the algorithm to recognize several specific features in more than one defined class, and then applying an SVM (or other classifier) to classify new objects.

Regression

Linear or logarithmic binomial regression models make a binary prediction of classification based on one or more features or predictors. Multinomials are used for multiple potential classes. Both evaluate the relationship between features and predict optimal classifications for each object. Dozens of specific regression techniques exist and the performance of each regression method depends largely on the image set and individual features being tested.[17]

Random Forest Classifiers

Finally, groups of classification and regression models can be combined to evaluate random features, rather than user-defined features, to predict the most accurate class for any object.[18]

In summary, statistical classification algorithms may be used in combination with each other or with traditional image segmentation methods to create classes of objects with like features. This is critical for segmenting and classifying tumor regions from stromal regions, nuclei from cytoplasms, or nucleoli within a nucleus.

FEATURE EXTRACTION, RESULT GENERATION, INTERPRETATION, AND REPORTING

Once an image has been accurately segmented and classified into its component parts of interest, for example, tumor and stroma or nuclei and cytoplasms, meaningful information may be extracted. The information that can be extracted should be directly relevant to the question being asked. For example, the size of nuclei may be important in classifying cancer nuclei, but may not be important when the question is the IHC intensity of the cancer nuclei. It is tempting to extract hundreds to thousands of features for every object (perhaps every cell); however, this may make it difficult to interpret and report meaningful findings.

Rather, the question and features should be directly linked. To quantify nuclear pleomorphism, a number of features of nuclear geometry may be useful: roundness, ellipticity, or circularity (which is mathematically different); however, texture or color features may not be directly relevant. That said, images that have been segmented and classified hold vast minable data. The number of data points for feature extractions of WSIs can easily exceed the volume of data produced by microarray and sequencing methods.

Results in any modern commercially available histologic image analysis product can be easily exported to standard file formats from .cvs to .xls or similar. It is highly recommended to engage a pathology informatics and/or biostatistician for in-depth interruptions of complex results. However, freeware and commercially available software can be used to interpret results and even help to identify how segmentation and classification methods can be improved to provide additional accuracy.

IMAGE ANALYSIS FOR BASIC AND TRANSLATIONAL RESEARCH USE

Image analysis is increasingly necessary for quantification of research projects. Surgical pathology research in particular has massive potential to transition from traditional qualitative and semi-quantitative methods of scoring and evaluating aspects of histologic tissues to repeatable quantifiable methodologies.

For example, IHC intensity and cellularity have been estimated by expert pathologists for decades using manual morphometric quantitative analysis. This is has been regarded as the gold standard in the field currently; however, it is generally realized that there is tremendous interobserver and intraobserver variability by manual method.[19–21] Increasingly, using image analysis technologies to quantifiably measure IHC intensity and cellularity provides for a more standardized, granular and repeatable measure of biological processes in tissue sections.[22] In this review, 2 main hypothetical and general examples of the utility of image analysis in research are discussed.

First, it can be recognized that novel biomarker discovery is becoming the focus of many international research programs. The fact that image analysis can be used to quantitatively evaluate novel biomarker staining intensity and patterning in large files and large sets of images is in itself very useful. Optimizing the throughput for pathologists performing research is a major advantage of image analysis; however, a more rapid scoring of samples may also be coupled with a more accurate determination of IHC intensity and localization in a more repeatable way. Furthermore, the nature of quantifiable values allows the user interpreting the results to have the confidence that all of the results were acquired with the exact same parameters making them directly comparable. Ideally, image analysis algorithms for research use should be tunable for different tissue types (eg, breast, lung, colon, prostate), different biomarkers (eg, ER, PR, HER2, Ki-67, P53, EGFR, CD117) and different reagents (immunohistochemical, chemical, and immunofluorescence).

Second, high-resolution data appropriate for computers (eg, color values from 0–255) may be requiring coarser stratification (eg, 0–3) for human interpretation. For example, if an investigator is interested in progression-free survival time as it relates to a specific biomarker, high-resolution data derived from the image analysis results can better separate the groups with long and short survival times.

Image analysis in research is undoubtedly driven by the promise of clinical relevance. Although histologic image analysis pendulum is hanging firmly on the research side of almost every institution, it is clear that it is moving toward clinical applications. For the purposes of this article a key group of image analysis applications, which are still in the research phase, hold great promise for clinical decision support. Some exemplary applications identified include the following:

1. The ability to accurately and reliably quantify the *area of tumor* on a slide by counting the number and measuring the size of tumor cells in a WSI[23]
2. The measure of *immunologic response* to a disease by coupling digital pathology, image analysis, and immunoscore metrics[24]
3. Analysis for diagnosis, prognosis, and prediction of therapy[25–27]
4. Mitotic activity and proliferation index, such as mitotic count, PHH3, and Ki-67[28–30]
5. *Nuclear feature* quantification[31]
6. A deeper interrogation of the *tumor microenvironment* and tumor-to-stroma interface[32]
7. *Tumor necrosis* quantification[33]
8. Automated assistance with the high-throughput applications of *tissue microarray slides*[34]
9. Interrogating tumor heterogeneity[35]
10. Immunofluorescent applications quantification, multiplexing, unmixing, and fluorescence in situ hybridization or in situ hybridization applications [22,35]

IMAGE ANALYSIS FOR CLINICAL USE

Although image analysis for research use in surgical pathology is increasing in scope and in breadth at a rapid pace, clinical use of image analysis is limited to a few key algorithms approved by the Food and Drug Administration (FDA). The first commercially available FDA-cleared algorithms for clinical use originated about a decade ago. Since then, little advancement has been made in the field. The currently available image analysis algorithms approved for clinical use include the IHC quantification of estrogen receptor, progesterone receptor, HER2, p53, and Ki-67. There are 2 FDA-approved platforms intended for use as aid to the pathologist in detection and quantification of biomarkers of breast cancer; however, in one system, the biomarkers, scanners, digital reading, and image analysis algorithms have been optimized and clinically validated to work as a cohesive system. In another system, the reading of digital IHC slides from a computer monitor was first cleared by the FDA, while image analysis application received FDA approval later. In addition, the application can be independently tuned or adjusted to accommodate a laboratory's unique staining process.

In general, FDA clearance encompasses a complete digital pathology system, including scanners for creating digital slide images from microscope slides; digital pathology information management system for managing, viewing, and analyzing digital slides; and the specific image analysis application that performs the automated scoring of biomarkers. Currently, the need for extremely robust algorithm precision has limited the scope of image analysis in anatomic pathology to IHC intensity and localization quantification. Although the promise of using image analysis to enhance the clinical workflow in anatomic pathology is sure to become a reality, the timeline of this transition remains unpredictable.

SUMMARY

Image analysis has been refining the course of anatomic pathology for decades. It provides a new avenue for a more rapid and accurate interrogation of WSIs and has been accelerating significantly in maturation over the past 10 years. Image analysis allows pathologists to work in a more quantitative and repeatable way. It can be used to provide information more rapidly and enhance the pathology workflow. The adoption of image analysis in pathology also continues to increase as digital pathology becomes more commoditized and common in pathology departments worldwide.

REFERENCES

1. Serra J. Image analysis and mathematical morphology, vol. 1. London: Academic Press; 1982.
2. Duncan JS, Ayache N. Medical image analysis: progress over two decades and the challenges ahead. IEEE Trans Pattern Anal Mach Intell 2000; 22(1):85–106.
3. Lloyd MC, Allam-Nandyala P, Purohit CN, et al. Using image analysis as a tool for assessment of prognostic and predictive biomarkers for breast cancer: How reliable is it? J Pathol Inform 2010;1:29.
4. Meijer GA, Belien JA, Van Diest PJ, et al. Origins of... image analysis in clinical pathology. J Clin Pathol 1997;50(5):365–70.
5. Horowitz SL, Pavlidis T. Picture segmentation by a directed split-and-merge procedure In: Proceedings of the Second International Joint Conference on Pattern Recognition, vol. 424. San Rafael, CA: Morgan & Claypool; 1974. p. 433.
6. Finkel RA, Bentley JL. Quad trees: a data structure for retrieval on composite keys. Acta Inform 1974; 4(1):1–9.
7. Jiang X, Mojon D. Adaptive local thresholding by verification-based multithreshold probing with application to vessel detection in retinal images. IEEE Trans Pattern Anal Mach Intell 2003;25(1): 131–7.

8. Tek FB, Dempster AG, Kale I. Blood cell segmentation using minimum area watershed and circle radon transformations. In: Ronse C, Najman L, Decencière E, editors. Mathematical morphology: 40 years on. Springer Netherlands; 2005. p. 441–54.

9. Filipczuk P, Kowal M, Obuchowicz A. Automatic breast cancer diagnosis based on K-means clustering and adaptive thresholding hybrid segmentation. In: Choraś, Ryszard S, editors. Image processing and communications challenges 3. Springer Berlin Heidelberg; 2011. p. 295–302.

10. Lee J, Haralick RM, Shapiro LG. Morphologic edge detection. IEEE J Robot Autom 1987;3(2):142–56.

11. Meyer-Baese A, Schmid VJ. Pattern recognition and signal analysis in medical imaging. Oxford, UK: Elsevier; 2014.

12. Kandemir M, Feuchtinger A, Walch A, et al. Digital pathology: multiple instance learning can detect Barrett's cancer. Beijing, China: ISBI; 2014.

13. Cruz-Roa A, Basavanhally A, González F, et al. Automatic detection of invasive ductal carcinoma in whole slide images with convolutional neural networks. In: Gurcan MN, Madabhushi A, editors. SPIE medical imaging. International Society for Optics and Photonics; 2014. p. 904103.

14. Bioucas-Dias J, Condessa F, Kovacevic J. Alternating direction optimization for image segmentation using hidden Markov measure field models. In: Gurcan MN, Madabhushi A, editors. IS&T/SPIE electronic imaging. International Society for Optics and Photonics; 2014. p. 90190P.

15. Zhang G, Yin J, Su X, et al. Augmenting multi-instance multilabel learning with sparse Bayesian models for skin biopsy image analysis. Biomed Res Int 2014;2014:305629.

16. Ishikawa T, Takahashi J, Takemura H, et al. Gastric lymph node cancer detection using multiple features support vector machine for pathology diagnosis support system. In: Goh, James, editors. The 15th International Conference on Biomedical Engineering. Singapore: Springer International Publishing; 2014. p. 120–3.

17. Yeh F-C, Ye Q, Kevin Hitchens T, et al. Mapping stain distribution in pathology slides using whole slide imaging. J Pathol Inform 2014;5:1.

18. Rexhepaj E, Brennan DJ, Holloway P, et al. Novel image analysis approach for quantifying expression of nuclear proteins assessed by immunohistochemistry: application to measurement of oestrogen and progesterone receptor levels in breast cancer. Breast Cancer Res 2008;10(5):R89.

19. Glatz K, Pritt B, Glatz D, et al. A multinational, Internet-based assessment of observer variability in the diagnosis of serrated colorectal polyps. Am J Clin Pathol 2007;127(6):938–45.

20. Karabulut A, Reibel J, Hamilton Therkildsen M, et al. Observer variability in the histologic assessment of oral premalignant lesions. J Oral Pathol Med 1995; 24(5):198–200.

21. Robertson AJ, Anderson JM, Swanson Beck J, et al. Observer variability in histopathological reporting of cervical biopsy specimens. J Clin Pathol 1989;42(3): 231–8.

22. Rojo MG, Bueno G, Slodkowska J. Review of imaging solutions for integrated quantitative immunohistochemistry in the pathology daily practice. Folia Histochem Cytobiol 2010;47(3):349–54.

23. Sherwin JC, Mirmilstein G, Pedersen J, et al. Tumor volume in radical prostatectomy specimens assessed by digital image analysis software correlates with other prognostic factors. J Urol 2010;183(5): 1808–15.

24. Anitei MG, Zeitoun G, Mlecnik B, et al. Prognostic and predictive values of the immunoscore in patients with rectal cancer. Clin Cancer Res 2014;20(7):1891–9.

25. Helm J, Centeno BA, Coppola D, et al. Histologic characteristics enhance predictive value of American Joint Committee on Cancer staging in resectable pancreas cancer. Cancer 2009;115(18):4080–9.

26. Kayser K, Görtler J, Bogovac M, et al. AI (artificial intelligence) in histopathology–from image analysis to automated diagnosis. Folia Histochem Cytobiol 2010;47(3):355–61.

27. Sarode VR, Han JS, Morris DH, et al. A comparative analysis of biomarker expression and molecular subtypes of pure ductal carcinoma in situ and invasive breast carcinoma by image analysis: relationship of the subtypes with histologic grade, Ki67, p53 overexpression, and DNA ploidy. Int J Breast Cancer 2011;2011:217060.

28. Fasanella S, Leonardi E, Cantaloni C, et al. Proliferative activity in human breast cancer: Ki-67 automated evaluation and the influence of different Ki-67 equivalent antibodies. Diagn Pathol 2011; 6(Suppl 1):S7.

29. Fujimori Y, Fujimori T, Imura J, et al. An assessment of the diagnostic criteria for sessile serrated adenoma/polyps: SSA/Ps using image processing software analysis for Ki67 immunohistochemistry. Diagn Pathol 2012;7:59.

30. Lee LH, Yang H, Bigras G. Current breast cancer proliferative markers correlate variably based on decoupled duration of cell cycle phases. Sci Rep 2014;4:5122.

31. Landini G, Rippin JW. Quantification of nuclear pleomorphism using an asymptotic fractal model. Anal Quant Cytol Histol 1996;18(2):167–76.

32. Rejniak KA, Estrella V, Chen T, et al. The role of tumor tissue architecture in treatment penetration and efficacy: an integrative study. Front Oncol 2013;3:111.

33. Lloyd MC, Alfarouk KO, Verduzco D, et al. Vascular measurements correlate with estrogen receptor status. BMC Cancer 2014;14(1):279.

34. Nocito A, Kononen J, Kallioniemi OP, et al. Tissue microarrays (TMAs) for high-throughput molecular pathology research. Int J Cancer 2001;94(1): 1–5.

35. Faratian D, Christiansen J, Gustavson M, et al. Heterogeneity mapping of protein expression in tumors using quantitative immunofluorescence. J Vis Exp 2011;56:e3334.

Printed and bound by CPI Group (UK) Ltd, Croydon, CR0 4YY

03/10/2024

01040384-0006